# Contents

# Contents

# Family therapy

**Library of Social Work**

General Editor:
Noel Timms
Professor of Social Work Studies
University of Newcastle upon Tyne

# Family therapy

# The treatment of natural systems

**Sue Walrond-Skinner**
*Principal Family Therapist*
*The Family Institute, Cardiff*

**Routledge & Kegan Paul**
London, Henley and Boston

First published in 1976
by Routledge & Kegan Paul Ltd
39 Store Street,
London WC1E 7DD,
Broadway House,
Newtown Road,
Henley-on-Thames,
Oxon RG9 1EN and
9 Park Street,
Boston, Mass. 02108, USA
Set in 10 on 11pt English
and printed in Great Britain by
The Lavenham Press Limited
Lavenham, Suffolk

ISBN 0 7100 8325 4 (c)
ISBN 0 7100 8326 2 (p)

# Preface

Despite the ever increasing American literature on family therapy, there has as yet been little writing on the subject produced in this country. In part, this reflects family therapy's more recent adoption in Britain, for it has only gradually begun to be incorporated into most social workers' repertoire of skills. There are still only a few professional training courses for social work students which offer systematic teaching in family therapy, even as an optional extra. But the number is increasing each year, and the growing interest in this treatment method is shown by the now frequent demands for more training opportunities and by the enthusiastic response with which study conferences on family therapy have been greeted during the last few years.

The chief purpose of this book is to provide a simple text describing the theoretical underpinnings of family therapy and some techniques of treatment which the method proposes. Considerable use has been made of case illustrations and wherever possible, verbatim transcripts of interviews have been used, to try to demonstrate some of the minute by minute flow of a family therapy session. Although the book is written primarily for social workers, it is hoped that those employed in other branches of the helping professions such as psychiatry, general medicine, clinical psychology and counselling may find the book useful as an introduction to this method of therapeutic intervention.

This book has emerged from my ongoing practice of family therapy at the Family Institute, Cardiff and from my teaching commitment to social work students at the Institute, and to post-graduate training courses for professional workers in the various fields of mental health. These, my colleagues, and the families with which I have worked have written the book: I have simply put it together.

# Preface

I can only pay acknowledgment to a few of those who have assisted more directly in the preparation of this book and I do so gratefully as follows: To the Family Institute, Cardiff, which has provided so much of the material for this book and especially to my colleagues, Dr Harvey Jones, Mr Brian Cade, Mrs Emilia Dowling and Dr Evan Davies; to the student members of the Institute, too numerous to mention by name; and to the families with whom I have had the privilege of working. My special thanks are due to Mr Brian Cade for supplying the illustrations; to Dr Barnardo's and its staff, who took the initial risk of supporting the Family Institute and who have so generously fostered it during its infancy and who continue to do so now in its later development; to the staff of the N.W. Ackerman Family Institute, New York, who cared for me, taught me and continue to enrich me with their friendship and wisdom, especially to the Director, Dr Don Bloch and to Dr Kitty La Perriere, Director of Education; to those connected with the Family Programme in the Department for Children and Parents at the Tavistock Clinic, London, who have offered much informal stimulation and help; to Dr Mary Essex for her encouragement and support during the early stages of the Family Institute's existence; to the Editor, for his helpful and constructive suggestions made throughout the preparation of the text; to Miss Myra James and her staff, for supervising the typing of the manuscript with such care, patience and good humour; to my valued friend and colleague, Di Johnson, for her continual encouragement and enthusiasm, when mine was in danger of flagging. Last, and most importantly, to the members of my own family, who I am gradually beginning to know afresh.

# Chapter one

# Introduction

Heaven and earth and I are of the same root,
The ten thousand things and I are of one substance.

Sojo, A Zen Monk Scholar

## Definitions

Family therapy can be defined as the psychotherapeutic treatment
of a natural social system, the family, using as its basic medium,
conjoint interpersonal interviews. Two parallel post-war developments have led to its appearance in the repertoire of psychotherapeutic treatment approaches in recent years. In the United
States, a new emphasis on social psychology, characterised by a
shift from the individual unit to groups and to larger networks,
coincided with the birth of a new field of technology surrounding
the development of computers, deriving from the science of
systems analysis and the theory of communications. These
seemingly unrelated developments contributed to an intellectual
climate in which the psycho-social *environment* or *context* in
which human beings lived began to attract the attention of
clinicians. The shift in interest in the United States from the
*individual* to the *individual as a function of his psycho-social
context,* was paralleled in England by the writings of phenomen-
ological thinkers and existentialist philosophers, poets and
clinicians. These developments, cutting across disciplines on both
sides of the Atlantic, led to a radically altered conception of the
human condition and of the nature of change. One could perhaps
summarise this altered conception, which forms the philosophical
base line of family therapy, by saying that its concern is with the
interdependence of seemingly opposing entities—unit and context,
sickness and health, part and whole, deviant and normal,
individual and community. This view of society is at variance with

1

society's own need to project on to the few the sick, mad and bad parts of itself—a need which is mirrored in microcosm by the society of the family, which so often isolates its deviance and dysfunction within one single member. Both the macrocosm (society) and the microcosm (the family) enable madness to remain outside the Self by locking it safely within the Other. Just as part of the concern of Laing, Szasz and their followers is with the healthy sanity of madness as an inner experience which can even be of value to the Self and the Self's Others in society, part of the family therapist's concern is with the therapeutic potential of persons who have become labelled sick or deviant members of their family groups. Thus, family therapy can be viewed as a clinical expression of a much larger movement which has influenced and been influenced by developments in such diverse fields as philosophy, political thought, literature, cybernetics, anthropology and sociology, as well as by the older methods of psychotherapy.

## Historical development and current status

Family therapy, which began hesitantly in American psychiatric and social work circles in the 1950s, reached major proportions by the late 1960s. In 1970, it merited the attention of the Group for the Advancement of Psychiatry, when family therapy was the subject of its annual report. With the help of an increasing range of detailed and varied literature; with the setting up of specialist agencies to practise family therapy and to train students; and with the inauguration of regular conferences and workshops devoted to different aspects of this treatment method, family therapy has now taken firm root in the American psychiatric and social work professions.

Historically, Britain can lay claim to an early interest in the idea of treating the family as a group. Social workers, before being overtaken by the American concentration on psycho-analytically oriented casework, had shown considerable interest in the systemic properties of families, sometimes adopting the practice of seeing groups of family members together, as a natural and obvious way of working. In non-clinical circles too, the simultaneous treatment of family members, and the relationship between them, was already beginning to emerge.

In his play *The Cocktail Party*, first published in 1940, T. S. Eliot describes an early attempt to offer conjoint marital therapy, together with the reaction of the patient to the unusualness of this procedure!

REILLY
Before I treat a patient like yourself
I need to know a great deal more about him,

Than the patient himself can always tell me.
Indeed, it is often the case that my patients
Are only pieces of a total situation
Which I have to explore. The single patient
Who is ill by himself, is rather the exception.
I have recently had another patient
Whose situation is much the same as your own.
You must accept a rather unusual procedure:
I propose to introduce you to the other patient.

> EDWARD

What do you mean? Who is this other patient?
I consider this very unprofessional conduct—
I will not discuss my case before another patient.

> REILLY

On the contrary. That is the only way
In which it can be discussed. . . . . .
    (LAVINIA is shown in by the NURSE-SECRETARY)
But here is the other patient.

> LAVINIA

Well, Sir Henry!
I said I would come to talk about my husband:
I didn't say I was prepared to meet him.

> EDWARD

And I did not expect to meet *you*, Lavinia,
I call this a very dishonourable trick.

> REILLY

Honesty before honour, Mr. Chamberlayne.
Sit down, please, both of you.

But 1951 marks a particularly important historical moment in the growth of family therapy. In a much described encounter in London, Dr John Sutherland from the Tavistock Clinic, London, and Dr John Bell from the Mental Research Institute, Palo Alto, discussed Dr John Bowlby's work and the therapeutic possibilities of seeing whole families together. In fact, as the story goes, Dr Bell misunderstood the technique being used by Dr Bowlby—who at that time was not undertaking the treatment of whole family groups—but out of this misunderstanding was born John Bell's early experimental work with family group therapy, which in turn influenced other clinicians in the development of its practice (Bell, 1961).

At present, however, we seem somewhat ambivalent in this country about the use of family therapy. The slowly growing interest in this treatment method during the last ten years has been overtaken before it has been even fully awakened, by newer develop-

3

ments still. Community work, direct political action to modify the social environment, and an urgent concern with clients' welfare rights, have all shown themselves to be effective methods of social work intervention.

At the same time, practitioners and teachers of these methods have challenged the appropriateness of casework intervention and have directed a similar challenge to family therapy, viewing it as a branch of the casework 'tree' rather than as a distinct method in its own right. As a result, there seems to be a danger that family therapy will be swept away as irrelevant or 'precious' before social workers in this country have had sufficient opportunity to examine its potential for themselves.[1] This would be unfortunate, for family therapy has much to offer the social work profession as well as the families for whom it cares: family therapy is in itself a bridging concept, both between different methods of social work intervention and between the helping professions themselves. Family therapy is concerned with the community of the family group and with the tensions and pain of co-existence in that group—just as community work's focus is the interlocking tensions of a more complex, but basically similar sort of system. On the other hand, the techniques of family therapy are sufficiently refined to make use of the shared conscious and unconscious intra-psychic levels of family life and to work with these at a depth which is normally assumed to be possible only when undertaking psycho-analytically oriented casework or psychotherapy.

**Interdisciplinary ethos**

As a means of forming links between social work and the other helping professions, family therapy has a special place. The method was conceived by and born into an interdisciplinary family, and its youthful development continues to be nurtured and enriched by practitioners from psychiatry, social work and psychology. It is through their care and concern for this common child that these different disciplines can be brought closer together as co-equal partners, respecting each other's different backgrounds, but recognising in family therapy, a common field of practice. This interdisciplinary ethos has remained a hallmark of the method, and springs from the therapeutic focus on the whole family system. If the family as a whole is to be treated, no place is left for the fragmentation of skills whereby a psychiatrist treats the child, a social worker visits the parents, and a psychologist is confined entirely to the role of diagnostician. Thus the way is opened up for the development of a more sophisticated interdisciplinary support system.

4

## Comparisons with other social work methods

Family therapy is not synonymous with 'family casework', nor with 'the family approach'—an even less specific phrase. The family approach has been used by practitioners from all disciplines; in fact few would claim intentionally to disregard the family in their therapeutic work, though many would admit that they are forced to do so in practice. But clearly, it is in no sense true to say that paying attention to the client's family is new. Family relationships have provided a rich *diagnostic* aid to the clinician for years, enabling him to obtain a much fuller picture of his client's difficulties. For example, within the psycho-analytic movement Johnson and Szurek (1952), using collaborative therapy in the 1940s, noted the concept of interlocking pathology between parent and child—with the child acting out the parents' forbidden impulses. The concept of the schizophrenogenic mother is another familiar example, where the aetiology of schizophrenia was viewed as involving the relationship between mother and child (Reichard and Tillman, 1950). These approaches had in common the fact that they were concerned only with a specific relationship within the family group and always one which involved the identified patient in an apparently obvious way. Gradually, this practice of observing the client's relatives for a fuller and more informed diagnosis, became well established. More rarely, the family has been actively involved by the clinician in the *treatment* process—but this too is not new. All who are familiar with Freud's account (1909) of his treatment of little Hans's phobia, using Hans's father as the therapist, will be aware of how far back one can trace the direct therapeutic use of clients' relatives, a practice which has been continued and developed by those who practise parental and marital behaviour modification (Hawkins *et al.,* 1971). Such practitioners, in common with most family caseworkers, have used the family *instrumentally* in both their diagnostic and their therapeutic work, as a means of assisting change within individual family members.

But family therapy as a distinctive treatment method must be defined much more closely and specifically. If we consider four important aspects of any therapeutic contract, we can begin to see how family therapy differs from both individual work and from group therapy. In individual treatment, communication occurs within a dyadic framework; treatment interventions are usually verbal; the major therapeutic focus is the intra-psychic life of the client and the primary therapeutic goal is growth of the individual. In group therapy, communication is interactional; treatment interventions are usually verbal; the major therapeutic focus is the group process and the primary therapeutic goal is growth of the individual in terms of his relationship with others. In all these aspects, family therapy differs significantly. Communication is transactional; treatment interventions are often non-verbal; the major therapeutic focus is the family system; and the primary therapeutic goal is change in the family's transactional system, rather than changes in the behaviour of its individual members. Thus, family therapy involves the treatment of the natural system itself; not the treatment of one or more of its components, nor the treatment of one part of the system by another. 'This goal of changing the family system of interaction is family therapy's most distinctive feature, its greatest advantage and, especially to those who come to it from other disciplines, its greatest stumbling block' (Beels and Ferber, 1969). Table 1.1, compares and contrasts family therapy with five other treatment methods available for use by social workers.

The family therapist does not use the family as an aid, however important, to arrive at a fuller diagnosis of the individual client's pathology, nor as a tool for more effectively treating the individual. The family therapist's task is not the manipulation of the family as a means of helping individual family members, but 'the transformation of the family into a more perfectly functioning group' (Bell, J. E., quoted in Beels and Ferber, 1969). It is this basic fact which, above all else makes family therapy a discontinuous development from individual treatment. It is the *family* who becomes the client for the family therapist, and this presents us with a conceptual leap that has the most significant consequences, both for techniques of intervention and for the outcome of treatment.

Family therapy is not only a technical approach towards treatment, however, it is also a theoretical view of pathology, giving rise to a whole range of treatment possibilities. Therapeutic interventions directed towards the primary family group, the marital dyad, the vertical and lateral kin networks, and to artificially formed groups of families all arise from the fundamental philosophical viewpoint that characterises family therapy, viz. the interdependence of family members' emotional, psychological and behavioural manifestations. Thus, conjoint marital therapy, network therapy, multiple family therapy and multiple impact therapy, are all sub-specialities of this one method of work. Because this is so, the approach, focus and therapeutic goal is identical in each. Table 1.2 sets out a comparison between them.

Looking at Table 1.2, it becomes clear that the family therapist's unit of treatment can be both broader and narrower than the nuclear family system. His treatment group, can, for example, consist of one person or of a group of perhaps forty people—if he is engaging in network therapy. His definition of 'family' does not rely primarily on ties of blood, but on ties of emotion, and his concern is

TABLE 1.1 Comparison of treatment interventions

| Therapeutic Unit | Individual | Individuals in an emotional relationship | Family Group | Group | Community | Institutional |
|---|---|---|---|---|---|---|
| Method | Individual psychotherapy Psycho-analytically oriented casework | Family casework Collaborative marital or parent/child therapy Concurrent marital or parent/child therapy | Family therapy | Group work Group therapy Growth groups | Community work | Residential work Therapeutic communities |
| Approach | Intra-personal | Interpersonal | Transactional | Interactional | Interactional | Interactional |
| Focus | Intra-psychic | Interlocking | Family system | Group process | Inter-group process | Group and inter-group process |
| Goal | Growth of individual | Growth within the particular relationship being treated | Higher degree of functioning in the family system | Growth of self in relationship to others | Improvement and change in community inter-group relationships | Growth of self in relationships and improvement of inter-group relations |

TABLE 1.2  Sub-specialities of family therapy

| Therapeutic Unit | Individual | Individuals in an emotional relationship | Family Group | Group | Community | Institutional |
|---|---|---|---|---|---|---|
| Method | 1 Individual work with a 'healthy' family member<br>2 Individual work with identified patient | 1 Conjoint marital therapy<br>2 Conjoint parent/child therapy<br>3 Conjoint work with other emotional relationships | Conjoint family therapy | Multiple family therapy and Multiple couples therapy (non-residential) | Network therapy | 1 Multiple impact therapy<br>2 Multiple family therapy |
| Approach | Intra-personal and transactional | Transactional | Transactional | Interactional and transactional | Transactional | Interactional and transactional |
| Focus | Operative system | Operative system | Operative system | Operative system | Operative system | Operative system |
| Goal | Higher degree of functioning in the family system | Higher degree of functioning in the family system | Higher degree of functioning in the family system | Higher degree of functioning in the family system | Higher degree of functioning in the family system | Higher degree of functioning in the family system |
| Diagnostic Indicator | 1 Lack of motivation on part of other members—or as a means of gaining purchase on a deadlocked system<br>2 When treatment goal is separation from family, as with adolescent problems (Undertaken as *additional* to other systems therapy) | 1 Childless marital system or work with this sub-system as part of programme of treatment of whole family<br>2 Single parent families<br>3 Common law marriages; homosexual couples; stable friendship systems | When the family is the significant container of dysfunction | Isolated family units. Family units which are too threatened to receive a therapist. Families where treatment can be accelerated when opportunities for identification with other similar families are given | 1 When extended family and/or neighbours, friends, are the significant container of dysfunction<br>2 Group of families living together communally | When it is helpful to provide the security of an institutional setting to accomplish rapid or prolonged change in family unit or in group of family units |

8

to engage the operative emotional system in treatment. Family therapy can, therefore, more accurately be described as systems therapy, since the term 'family' carries with it various connotations of boundary which do not necessarily relate to the boundary of the operative emotional system. A chart of the sub-specialities is given in order to indicate the breadth and potential of this method of work, and although this book is chiefly concerned with the principles and practice of the basic method, the use made of these sub-specialities by different practitioners will be touched upon briefly in chapter 9.

Returning to the chart of treatment interventions listed in Table 1.1, it is clear that family therapy is only one method available for use by the social worker. It is not the *only* method of working with families—nor is it always the most *appropriate* method of helping a family in difficulties. This book is simply concerned to examine the theoretical base and some of the treatment techniques which family therapy, as one treatment modality among many, offers the social worker for consideration.

## Note

1 Family therapy's main critics in this country come from the universities. Thought-provoking critiques have been offered by Pearson (1974) and Jordan (1972), Chapter 1.

# Chapter two

# Theoretical frameworks I

All parts of the organism form a circle. Therefore, every part is both beginning and end.

Hippocrates

Being a relatively new method of intervention, family therapy is currently undergoing a period of rapid transition and development. In Bowen's (1971) phrase, it is in 'a healthy unstructured state of chaos'. Differing and even opposing views of both theory and practice exist amongst family therapists, which is not surprising in a field which is still so young and experimental. The 1970 report of the Group for the Advancement of Psychiatry listed the twenty-one most influential family therapists in the United States and the field is as yet governed and influenced mainly by these early charismatic figures. The list includes such diverse personalities as Nathan Ackerman, Virginia Satir, Don Jackson, Carl Whitaker, Salvador Minuchin, Walter Kempler and Murray Bowen. With the notable exceptions of Nathan Ackerman and Don Jackson, most of these are still practising and writing and maintaining their enormous contribution to the field. But second and third 'generations' of family therapists have also appeared—some of whom have helped to constitute 'schools' of therapy surrounding the first generation figures. Others, particularly those outside the United States, have formed new centres, where experimental work is being developed in many different directions.

When attempting to elucidate the theoretical base of family therapy, one is confronted with a 'collage' of theoretical standpoints, which do not as yet constitute any unified whole. However, the need to move away from the medical model which has dominated traditional forms of casework and psychotherapy, with its emphasis on the individual and on a straight linear progression of cause and effect, has made the construction of supporting theory a pressing necessity. Yet in 1970, the Group for the Advancement of Psychiatry's report showed at least half a dozen rather ill-defined sources, from which practitioners were deriving their theory of families and of family therapy. Currently, the conceptual framework underpinning family therapy continues to be a matter of some confusion and of considerable debate—the problem being chiefly focused around the difficulty of evolving a theory that is both 'pure' enough to be universal and yet is capable of application to the diversity of the clinical situation. It is therefore difficult to create a synthesis out of the welter of theoretical standpoints that exist; and even if one were to succeed in distilling a pure and all embracing theory of the family, such an attempt would necessarily involve a high level of abstraction. However, the most promising theoretical model proposed so far is that of general systems theory, and this chapter will therefore be concerned with outlining this theory, which seems to provide the most comprehensive framework from which to practise. Although the theory poses the family therapist with certain practical dilemmas in its application, it nevertheless provides him with a conceptual framework with which to oppose the medical model and to move from the individual into the family group. Chapter 3 will test out the traditional psycho-analytic model against this framework.

**General systems theory**

General systems theory was conceived by Ludwig von Bertalanffy in the 1940s, in order to provide a working model for conceptualising phenomena which did not lend themselves to explanation by the mechanistic reductionism of classical science. In particular, general systems theory seemed able to provide a unifying theoretical framework for both the natural and the social sciences, which needed to employ concepts such as organisation, wholeness and dynamic interaction, none of which lent itself easily to the methods of analysis employed by the pure sciences. Ackoff places systems theory in its developmental context when he states: 'The tendency to study systems as an entity rather than as a conglomeration of parts is consistent with the tendency in contemporary science no longer to isolate phenomena in narrowly confined contexts, but rather to open *interactions* for examination and to examine larger and larger slices of nature' (Ackoff, 1960, p. 29; italics mine).

A system has been defined by Hall and Fagen as a 'set of objects together with the relationships between the objects and between their attributes. The objects are the component parts of the system, the attributes are the properties of the objects and the relationships tie the system together'. In general systems theory, there exists the system, the system's environment (supra-system) and the system's components (sub-systems); and the theory is concerned with the description and exploration of the relationship between this hierarchy of interrelated systems. In Koestler's words (1964, p. 287): 'the functional units on every level of the hierarchy are double-faced as it were; they act as whole when facing downwards, as parts when facing upwards.' The following concepts comprise the basis of systems theory, and provide a framework for applying the theory to the family group.

## Wholeness

General systems theory (GST) states that a system is a whole and that its objects (or components) and their attributes (or characteristics) can only be understood as functions of the total system. A system is not a random collection of components, but an interdependent organisation in which the behaviour and expression of each component influences and is influenced by all the others. The concept of wholeness implies in turn the concept of non-summativity —in other words, the whole constitutes more than simply the sum of its parts. GST's interest lies in the transactional processes that take place *between* the components of a system and between their attributes. Put another way, it is impossible to gain a significant understanding of a system solely by reviewing its component parts and 'adding up' one's impression of these. The character of the system transcends the sum of its components and their attributes and belongs to a higher order of abstraction. It would not be possible to gain much understanding of chess, for example, simply by looking at the pieces; one would need to examine the game as a whole, and to take note of how the movement of one piece affects the position and meaning of every other piece on the board. Applied to the family group, the theorist is concerned with this quality of non-summativity, by which the nature of the transactional processes between family members transcends the activity of individual family members themselves when viewed in isolation. Applied to the family therapy situation, this quality of wholeness describes not only the family system—but the new whole of family group + family therapist—the therapeutic system.

A vital means of determining a system's identity is its boundary. It is the system's boundary which provides an interface, both with its external environment and with its own sub-systems, and which circumscribes its identity in space and time. An important aspect of the family therapist's task is to help to determine the boundary of the family system; unless he is able to get a correct understanding of where the system's boundary lies, he will fail to engage or maintain in treatment the operative family system *as a whole*. Ultimately, unless he can do so, he will not be treating the family system—but merely a random collection of its component parts. Having plotted the system's boundary correctly, the family therapist may *then* decide to work at the interface of one or more of its sub-systems, but he will always do so from within the context of the system as a whole.[1]

The character of a system is described by Hall and Fagen (1956, p. 23) as either open or closed:

Organic systems are *open*, meaning they exchange materials, energies or information with their environments. A system is *closed* if there is no import or export in any of its forms, such as information, heat, physical materials, etc., and therefore no change of components, an example being a chemical reaction taking place in a sealed insulated container.

Clearly, using this definition, all organic systems, whether biological or social, are open. However, when reviewing the application of GST to family and other social systems a more refined concept is required. Ackoff (1971, p. 84) comments: 'Because systems researchers have found such conceptualisations [open/closed] of relatively restricted use, their attention has increasingly focused on more complex and "realistic" open systems. "Openness" and "closedness" [are seen] *simultaneously* [as] properties of systems and our conceptualisations of them.' In other words, the concepts of closedness and openness can be seen as *relative* in the context of family and other social systems, and one can imagine a continuum moving from the relatively open family system, engaged in a high degree of communication with its supra-system (the community, the extended family, etc.) and between its sub-systems (individual members and sub-groupings); to the relatively closed family system, engaged in minimal interchange with either its suprasystem or with its sub-systems. Moreover, one cannot simply think of relatively open family systems as functional, and relatively closed family systems as dysfunctional. Jordan (1972) for example, has described two family types—the centrifugal family and the integrative family, where both the former (an open system) and the latter (a closed system) can be considered as being highly dysfunctional. Similarly, Minuchin (1974b) has described two broad family types as disengaged and enmeshed—the extreme points of each category being dysfunctional.

## Protection and growth

The concept of homeostasis (or morphostasis as it is sometimes called) preceded the formal development of systems theory, being defined in the 1920s by W. B. Cannon. It was incorporated into the systems frame of reference and remains an important concept, especially in the branch of systems theory known as cybernetics. Homeostasis can be defined simply as 'same state' and it is this quality which enables a system to remain stable and in a 'steady state' through time. Homeostasis is made possible by the use of information coming from the external environment and being incorporated into the system in the form of 'feedback'. Feedback triggers the system's 'regulator', which by altering the system's internal condition, maintains homeostasis. For example: a homeostatic mechanism will be sensitive to changes within the supra-system and will functionally ward off the danger of confusion or disintegration which this may hold for the system. A much used example of the way in which homeostasis works is that of a central heating system which maintains the house in a 'steady state' of warmth. It makes use of a thermostat which acts as a regulator, and which responds to feedback concerning the temperature in the supra-system outside the house. When the temperature outside the house drops, the thermostat acts to raise the lowered temperature inside the house correspondingly.

Almost from the beginning, controversy has surrounded this concept of homeostasis—Bertalanffy (1972), for example, in his later writings has suggested that systems theory must move 'beyond the homeostasis principle', particularly in its application to sociocultural systems. Many systems theorists have found that homeostasis is not a sufficiently comprehensive explanation for processes which operate in social systems, since it cannot explain phenomena such as growth, change and creativity. Homeostasis is a self-correcting mechanism. It is essentially concerned with the preservation of what is, against the onslaught of external stress factors; it cannot explain the propensity of higher organisms and well-functioning social systems to move on to higher orders of complexity. Two problems therefore confront the theorist in the extrapolation of the homeostasis principle to family therapy: first, the confusing tendency of some theorists to equate homeostasis with dysfunction; and second, the insufficiency of the concept in explaining some of the more complex phenomena of social and hence of family systems.

Unless one subscribes to the belief that constant revolution is the optimal condition of all social systems, there can be no simple equation between homeostasis and pathological rigidity. In correcting this idea, we are returning to a more accurate presentation of Cannon's (1939) original concept, whereby homeostasis was viewed as a functional, protective mechanism. Homeostasis 'does not imply something set and immobile, a stagnation. It means a condition—a condition which may vary, but which is relatively constant'. Clearly, the healthy, functional family system requires a measure of homeostasis in order to survive the 'slings and arrows of outrageous fortune', and to maintain stability and security within its physical and social environment. It is only when these mechanisms 'overfunction' that the system becomes fixed and dysfunctional in its rigidity. The solution to this dysfunctional activity is not the removal of the homeostatic regulator. If one were to remove the thermostat from a central heating system which was already overheating, the whole system (together with its immediate environment, the house) would probably blow up. A similar result is often witnessed when the identified patient or family 'regulator' is removed to hospital, prison or children's home, or is successfully treated via individual psychotherapy or casework. The identified person improves dramatically, but the family collapses. (Families, of course, often intuitively perceive the dangers to their structure of the caseworker's efforts to alter the individual, and, whilst verbally protesting their desire for the identified patient's well-being, they make strenuous efforts to prevent his improvement.) If the family is unsuccessful in resisting the caseworker's efforts to render its regulator inactive, another alternative open to it is decompensation by another family member. In other words, another member must be designated as the 'family regulator'.

Homeostatic mechanisms are therefore required in both adequately and inadequately functioning systems and their removal brings about catastrophe in either type of circuit. The same applies to the family, which, as a system, requires either inter-personal or intra-personal homeostatic mechanisms in order to operate effectively.

The following example illustrates the functional and dysfunctional operation of homeostatic mechanisms. A family is faced with several external threats to its survival, such as an acute physical illness in mother and unemployment in father. Mother has to be hospitalised for a period and father has to find a new job. The family would need the assistance of homeostatic mechanisms to 'regulate' it in this crisis situation and might, for example, require the eldest daughter to take over some of mother's practical and emotional functions during her absence. She might need to be more 'maternal' to her younger siblings and more supportive and companionable to her father in his own insecurity. In this situation, the daughter's role changes would act as useful homeostatic mechanisms. However, if, when mother returned to health and father became well established in his new job, difficulties began to appear in the marital relationship, these original homeostatic mechanisms, far from alleviating the new problem, might well create secondary problems in themselves. Unfortunately, however, because the daughter's role changes had proved a useful means of combating the original external threats posed to the family system, the homeostatic mechanisms might actually start to *overfunction*. Rather than returning to her previous emotional position within the family and allowing father and mother to re-integrate their relationship as husband and wife, the daughter becomes agoraphobic, refusing to relinquish her role as 'mother' and 'housewife' and continuing to replace mother as father's constant companion and support. In this situation, the daughter, as an agoraphobic identified patient, then puts up a smokescreen in front of the marital relationship and, by concentrating the family's energy and attention on herself, she, on the one hand, prevents the marital difficulties from becoming explosive, but also prevents husband and wife from working on their difficulties in a way which could bring about some fundamental resolution. Wertheim (1973, p. 365) has suggested the use of two different terms as a way of clarifying this two-fold action of homeostasis (morphostasis): consensual morphostasis and forced morphostasis.

> *Consensual morphostasis* derives from appropriately balanced, intra-family distribution of power. The term refers to *genuine stability* of the family system, consensually validated by its members. Forced morphostasis is rooted in intra-family power imbalance. The term . . . refers to *apparent stability* of the family system maintained in the absence of genuine, consensual validation by its members.

The second problem confronting the family theorist—that of the insufficiency of homeostasis as an explanatory concept, has led several writers to expand the theory, and Watzlawick (1968) and Speer (1970) have suggested modifications. Speer, following Buckley, and other writers, has developed the idea of morphogenesis or growth—a concept which he feels has been overlooked by the over-concentration of the early family therapists on homeostasis. In contrast to homeostasis which, as we have seen, is concerned with the protection of what is, morphogenic mechanisms are concerned with growth and change. A particular result of morphogenesis is an increase in differentiation in the system's component parts, whereby each is able to develop in its complexity whilst remaining in functional relationship with the whole. The emphasis is moved from the *self-correction* of homeostasis, to the *self-direction* of morphogenesis. Speer subsumes both concepts into the overall term 'viability', which he uses to describe the essential character of family and other social systems. He sets the different system types in relation to each other as follows (1970, p. 270):

While equilibrium is the fundamental principle of organic, chemical and mechanical systems; and homeostasis is the basic principle of lower and higher biological and organismic systems; viability with the implication of inherent capacities for growth and self-directed change is the criterion principle for social systems.

Viability thus describes a system which is capable of both homeostatic and morphogenic growth processes in varying degrees. The extent to which the family system is able to employ *both* types of mechanism appropriately, to further its own unique goals, is the extent to which it can be described as healthy and functional.

## Communication

Because systems theory is concerned with the interrelationship between system components and between systems and supra-systems, a great deal of emphasis is placed upon communication, i.e. on *how* the systems components interact. With the development of GST the idea of the distribution of fixed quantities of energy gave way to the concept of information exchange, as the transactional currency of the system's *modus operandi*. As we will see, whilst the notion of fixed energy outputs was found sufficient to explain the psychoanalytic model, the concept of information exchange has a much higher degree of adaptability to family theory and treatment. Information exchange implies the concept of a mutually affecting process between components and involves the notion of feedback. One can compare the two different concepts by imagining a chain along which a message is passed from A to B; from B to C; and from C to D. This would be the model for the movement of fixed energy quantities. In contrast, in the feedback model of information exchange, the chain would appear: A to B; $B_1$ to C; $C_1$ to D; $D_1$ to A; $A_1$ to $B_1$, etc. In this chain, each link is modified and hence changed by its interaction and this modification occurs in a circular process, known as a feedback loop. Ultimately the last point in the chain is 'fed back' to the first point, indicating the dynamic nature of the whole exchange. A spider paralysing a fly by its sting is involved in the process of passing a fixed quantity of energy from A to B; a jelly-fish stinging a human foot may participate in a feedback loop from A to $B_1$ and from $B_1$ (the stung foot) back to $A_1$ (in the form of a circle). In the first model the effect of A on B does not get re-incorporated into the $(A + B)$ system; whereas in the second, the message from the affected $B_1$ (output) gets re-incorporated into the $(A + B)$ system as feedback (input). In GST, transactions are therefore viewed as circular and as creating progressively more complex spirals of exchange. An example from one of Laing's poems

17

will illustrate the increasing complexity of feedback spirals in family systems (Laing, 1970).

Jill thinks Jack is mean and greedy
Jack thinks Jill is mean and greedy
the more Jill feels that Jack is mean
the more greedy Jack feels Jill to be
the more Jill feels Jack is greedy
the more mean Jack feels Jill to be
the more greedy Jack feels Jill to be
  the more mean Jill feels Jack to be
  the more mean Jill feels Jack to be
the more greedy Jack feels Jill to be
Jack feels Jill is greedy
       because Jill feels Jack is mean
Jill feels Jack is mean
   because Jack feels Jill is greedy
Jack feels Jill is mean
   because Jill feels Jack is greedy

Jill feels Jack is greedy
   because Jack feels Jill is mean
The more
   Jack feels Jill is mean to feel he is greedy
the more
   Jill feels Jack is mean
      to feel she is mean to feel he is greedy
      to feel she is mean

The more Jill feels Jack is mean
   to feel she is mean to feel he is greedy to feel
               she is mean
the more Jack feels Jill is mean
  to feel
     Jack is mean
      to feel she is mean
      to feel he is greedy
      to feel she is mean
because she does not give him what he wants.

In GST, feedback is considered to be either negative or positive. In both cases, there is a transfer function whereby input is converted into output, which in turn is re-introduced into the system as information about the output. In the case of negative feedback, this information is used by the system to trigger off its homeostatic mechanisms and acts as a means of decreasing the system's output deviation and thus maintaining its 'steady state'. In the case of positive feedback, information is used to trigger off morphogenic mechanisms leading to the upset of homeostasis and the movement towards growth and change. In other words, positive feedback is used to amplify output deviation. There is, of course, no simple correlation between either type of feedback and desirability. As in the case of homeostasis and its opposite, growth, it is the use which a family system makes of either type of feedback, which designates it as being either helpful or disruptive to the family's overall needs and purpose.

Viewed from the point of view of GST, a family that comes into treatment has suffered some form of breakdown in the functioning of its feedback processes—either in terms of its internal transactions between family members, or in terms of its external transactions with the outside world (extended family, neighbours, community)—or in both. At the risk of over-simplifying the situation, we can reduce dysfunctional communication patterns to three types: communication can be either *blocked, displaced* or *damaged*. With the first possibility, transactions between family members or between the family and the outside world, may have become reduced to the extremes of prolonged silence, withdrawal, isolation, or to the bizarre, written communication which may be the sole link between members of the same household for years on end. The possibility of growth and change is drastically reduced by the blocking off of feedback mechanisms. Silence and withdrawal is, of course, a form of communication—but when variety is reduced to this one type, communication channels have become severely blocked. A less extreme example of blocked internal communication is the family 'secret'. Usually, the only secret involved is the fact that nobody knows that everybody knows it. Family members are at pains to protect the 'secret' and collude with each other in their efforts to do so. Any diversionary tactic is useful in maintaining the secret—a particularly effective one being the heavy scapegoating of a marginally involved family member. Therefore, an early question for the family therapist to ask himself (and the family) is: 'What are you *not* talking about by concentrating on Johnny's misbehaviour?'

Displacement occurs through the eruption of symptomatology—the selection of the symptom and the symptom bearer becoming highly significant means of communication between family members. The symptom becomes a displaced means of communicating an important truth about the family group. The family therapist will therefore be interested in *which* symptom has been selected and *who* has chosen (and been chosen) to carry it. For example: a family consisting of husband, wife and two adopted teenagers (a girl and boy) come for help because the boy has been found exposing himself in public. Although he is seen individually by his probation officer for a considerable period of time, his behaviour only becomes understandable in terms of displaced communication, when it is discovered that sexual expression within the marital dyad has ceased and that the husband is impotent. The family therapist who uses GST as his theoretical framework, thus views symptoms in terms of their interpersonal message rather than their intra-psychic meaning.

Third, communication processes can be severely *damaged* within the system. One of the most important examples of damaged communication processes is the 'double bind', described originally by a group of researchers at Palo Alto, California, whose work proved to be extremely influential in assisting the development of family therapy.[2] These workers state that every communicated message has two levels, the report level which is concerned with the *information* being conveyed; and the metacommunicative level, which is concerned with conveying a message *about* the information. The two levels may be congruent or incongruent. For example: the mother who calls to her child who has just fallen over, 'Come here darling, and let me hold you', while looking angry and embarrassed, is communicating to her child in such a way that the meta-communicative message (expressed by her angry face) contradicts the reported message (which conveys a desire to comfort the child). The result of such contradictory messages is confusion and im-mobility: the child is left uncertain as to which level of his mother's message to respond. Similarly, the only course left open for a family member caught in this kind of damaged communication process over a prolonged period of time, may be a schizophrenic withdrawal into the florid world of picture language, where his confusion can be expressed without fear of attacking his attacker. Whilst the report level is usually conveyed by words, the metacommunicative level is often expressed non-verbally through gesture, facial expression, voice tone, posture, etc. For double binding communication to result in serious confusion and distress, it must take place within the context of a relationship which has significance for both parties. Family therapists who work from the 'communication model' developed by Jay Haley, Jackson, Satir, Watzlawick and others, obviously make these communication processes the central plank of both their theory and their treatment procedures, an important part of treatment involving the correction of dysfunctional communication patterns and the clarification of meaning.[3]

**Causality**

In the classical model of pure science, causality is understood as being linear. In any given situation, we are taught to understand the 'cause' of an 'effect' by altering the variables one at a time until we *isolate* what produces a particular event. Moreover, as Shands (1971) points out, the very constraints which verbal language itself imposes upon us, continually encourage us to regard the universe as being organised on a linear basis, 'in cause-and-effect patterns of general relevance'. However, if one is working from the premise that many significant aspects of the system can only be understood by examining the system as a *whole,* aetiology has to be considered from a different point of view. For example, a family may see Johnny and his delinquency as the 'cause' of their distress, forgetting that Johnny's stealing may be reactive to his mother's emotional absence, which may be reactive to her husband's harsh handling of Johnny . . . to take a very simple example. And yet, instinctively we learn, what GST formulates explicitly, that we do not find this neat, linear ordering of cause and effect in the world, except by imposing it artificially. In GST, causality is viewed as a circular process. It is, therefore, *ipso facto,* without beginning or end, and thus any attempt by the therapist to transfer responsibility for how the family's problem started from one part of the system to another, is as inappropriate as the family's own 'blame game', which focuses on the identified patient as the source of the difficulty. We begin to learn 'how close apparent opposites may be when we understand the basically circular nature of human experience' (Shands, 1971). Whilst in some treatment interventions, such as psycho-analysis, healing and change spring from insight gained into the early traumata of certain childhood events, healing and change in family therapy is considered to proceed chiefly from an examination of *how* the family system is operating currently and an understanding of the function which problems hold for the goal oriented processes of the system's current existence. Theoretically, the concept of linear causality implies that the aetiological line moves from past to present—hence the need to delve back to the beginning of that line of events in order to understand. When using the concept of circular causality, the 'here and now' is emphasised, for it is in the here and now that the whole circle can be seen in operation. It is not so much that 'the past is a foreign country—they do things differently there' (to use Leo's thought from *The Go-Between*); but simply that, like a spiral staircase, the present re-enacts the past in such a way that meaning can be sought within the boundaries of the system's *current* processes. The past becomes redundant, and ecology rather than genesis becomes the family therapist's point of departure.

## Purpose

Organic and social systems are always goal-oriented and purposive.

Whilst in classical science, entities are viewed as being understandable in terms of their existence rather than their purpose, GST identifies the importance of a system's goal and purpose in gaining an understanding of the way its processes operate. Furthermore, GST recognises the tendency of a system to struggle to remain in being, even when it has developed dysfunctionally, rather than to disintegrate and go out of existence as a system. (All who work with families will recognise this tendency to cling desperately to the *status quo* of current family structure, however painful it appears to be for the individual family members concerned.) Since families are social systems, they are by nature goal-oriented and purposeful. When the family therapist joins the family system he does so in order to assist in re-directing it towards the achievement of its own unique purpose. In principle there is no moral dilemma involved in the fact that the therapeutic system is goal-oriented, for, being a social system, it would be so by its nature.

The purposeful and ongoing nature of a system allows us to gain a clearer understanding of the nature of the term *transaction,* often used in the systems approach to family therapy in preference to the more general term *interaction.* In point of fact, the two terms are sometimes used interchangeably in the systems literature; however, some writers have attempted to differentiate them in a way which further clarifies the specific nature of a system. According to Olson (1970): 'Whereas the interaction framework deals with person to person interacts, transaction deals with the process of inter-relationships in a historical and relational context.' And Framo (1965) comments: 'transaction suggests the unitary nature of the phenomenon with all its circular relatedness within a situational system.' Hence, it is the quality of relatedness in an ongoing historical sense which characterises the unique communication processes of members of a system—and which are thus described as being *transactional.*

In this chapter, an attempt has been made to examine in detail the general systems framework of family therapy. Much of the rest of this book will draw heavily, although not exclusively, upon the many insights which this theory offers the family therapist. The following chapter will examine another series of theoretical concepts and look at the way in which these can be integrated within general systems theory.

**Notes**

1 Dr Skynner provides an interesting discussion of this concept as it relates to the family system and to other types of systems, see Skynner (1974).
2 See, for example, papers on the double bind theory by Bateson *et al.* (1956).
3 Foley (1974) provides a helpful description of the theoretical contributions made by the communicational theorists, Jackson, Haley and Satir, and the different emphasis placed by each (see chapter 7).

# Chapter three

# Theoretical frameworks II

Every member of a living organism or social body has the dual
attributes of 'wholeness' and 'partness'.

Koestler, *The Act of Creation*

## The psycho-analytic framework: integration of the two theoretical models

The psycho-analytic framework differs from GST in so far as it is
essentially directed towards the nature and operation of the individual. Its usefulness for family therapy theory is therefore
questionable. Since this book rests on the premise that the theory
and method of family therapy necessarily derives from the systems
framework, we shall be concerned in this chapter to determine the
extent to which the psycho-analytic model can be integrated within
the systems framework and in what respects, if any, it extends our
understanding of the treatment of family groups.

Armstrong (1971) likens the struggle of members of a professional
family to evolve new theoretical frameworks to that of the family
group's efforts to allow its members to differentiate themselves, to
develop and to grow. Historically, each professional and scientific
community has made use of a central orienting paradigm, such as
Einstein's theory of relativity, Darwin's theory of evolution or
Freud's theory of the structure and operation of the human mind,
from which to construct subsidiary theory and to develop working
hypotheses. At any one time, the main body of professional or
scientific opinion will subscribe to this orienting paradigm. Using an
experiment conducted by Bruner and Postman (1949), Armstrong
describes the way in which a professional or scientific community
reacts to the discovery of new information which does not fit into the
existing orienting paradigm. Twenty-eight students were asked to

describe what they saw when playing cards were flashed on to a screen one at a time. The orienting paradigm was the fact that a pack of cards consists of four suits, two black (spades and clubs) and two red (diamonds and hearts). However, some of the cards shown to the students, such as a red six of spades, a black three of hearts, etc., did not fit into this paradigm. Bruner and Postman observed several interesting reactions to these anomalous cards. Some of the subjects refused the evidence of their own eyes and 'converted' the red spade to black in their description, to enable it to remain congruent with the orienting paradigm: in other words, they refused to recognise the card's incongruency. Others described the card as 'purplish, greyish, greenish, etc.' and, whilst recognising the card's incongruency, they tried to 'make it fit' into their conceptual framework. Still others became bewildered, confused and angry, and found it impossible to give a description of the card. A fourth group accurately described the six of spades as red, the three of hearts as black, etc. In other words, this fourth group was prepared to relinquish its allegiance to the orienting paradigm which stated that spades are black and hearts are red. These four responses are analogous to the way in which professional groups deal with data which cannot be assimilated into their prevailing frame of reference —deny the incongruency (analogous to Wynne's (*et al.* 1958) concept of pseudo-mutuality between family members); strait-jacket the data into the orienting paradigm, compromising both in the process; give up the whole endeavour in rage and confusion; or recognise the dilemma and record both the data *and* its incongruency, *vis-à-vis* the orienting paradigm. From this fourth response emerges the possibility of a creative synthesis between old and new, as well as the development of novel orienting paradigms.

Applied to the current position of family theory, many practitioners who have previously subscribed to the psycho-analytic framework, have responded to the development of a systems approach to families in one of three ways. First, by ignoring the challenge which it poses ('there is nothing new here—the red six of spades is black really'). Second, by strait-jacketing the psychotherapy of the family group wholesale into a psycho-analytic mould, and continuing to employ treatment techniques used in work with individuals. Third, by abandoning the whole idea of treating family groups because of the *impossibility* of strait-jacketing family treatment into the psycho-analytic framework and hence being fearful of alloying 'the pure gold' of psycho-analysis with the 'base metal' of the transactional approach. Thus, it is tempting for those who subscribe to the psycho-analytic model (and the training of most caseworkers is still heavily dependent on this model) to deal with the anomalous insights provided by GST by either 'ignoring, transforming or actively suppressing them' (Armstrong, 1971). On the other hand, it is equally tempting for the protagonists of GST to do likewise concerning psycho-analytic theory.

## Distinguishing features of the two theories

It seems to me that when confronted by these two frameworks and their respective claims to the position of orienting paradigm *vis-à-vis* our understanding and therapeutic management of families, our most constructive response is to recognise that there are areas both of incongruency and of synthesis between them.

As theoretical harmony can, I believe, only be sought *after* real differentiation has been achieved, I shall look first at what strike me as irreconcilable points of difference between the two theories, and their application in clinical practice. The first obvious point of departure is that the unit for psycho-analytic treatment interventions is the individual—in varying degrees of isolation from his psycho-social environment. It is of course true that, during his lifetime, Freud moved away from a strictly biological starting point, to an appreciation of the importance of social and cultural factors. Moreover, the 'neo-Freudians' such as Horney, Fromm and Harry Stack Sullivan, elaborated much more fully the importance of socio-cultural factors within the framework of psycho-analysis. Winnicott took these ideas even further when he began to conceive of the mother/child relationship as a social organism in itself. But all these developments are different from systems theory's concept of *wholeness*—involving as it does *the treatment of the natural system itself*. The appreciation which some present day psycho-analysts may have of the influence of a patient's family on pathology and on the treatment process is obviously significantly different from Freud's attitude to his patients' relatives: 'The most urgent warning I have to express is against any attempt to engage the confidence or support of parents and relatives . . . . The interference of relatives in psycho-analytical treatment is a very great danger, a danger one does not know how to meet' (1912, p. 333).

The analytic movement has developed a long way from this position but even so it has not made the conceptual leap required of the family therapist to the systems concept of 'wholeness'. Second, the psycho-analytic framework adopts the medical model's view that the objective expert must first diagnose the patient's illness (i.e. 'find its cause') and then prescribe suitable treatment. As Laing (1971b) points out: 'The hunt for the pathology "and the etiology of the disease" goes on, as much by those concerned with psychopathology as by those concerned with physical pathology.' But both the orderly progression in time from diagnosis to treatment (from 'cause' to 'effect') and the notion that the worker, whether analyst or caseworker, can remain outside either the diagnostic or the treatment procedure is at variance with GST's view of the non-summativity of a system's parts, which include both family members *and* family therapist as dynamic parts of the new whole of the treatment situation. The efforts of the analyst (and to a lesser degree, the analytically oriented caseworker) to remove 'contamination' from the therapeutic relationship by screening out many of his 'real' human responses to the patient or client is incompatible with a transactional view of human relationships—either inside or outside the treatment situation. As Yalom (1970) points out: in family therapy 'the therapist is defrocked, the therapeutic process is demystified'. Third, the psycho-analytic view of the nature of change is quite different from that of GST. Psycho-analytic treatment seeks to bring about change in a client by enabling him to gain insight into the reasons for his behaviour. Depending upon the particular school of psycho-analysis being followed, insight into the remote (Freud) or extremely remote (Klein) roots of traumata, the release of repressed feelings surrounding these events and the working through of the emotional tensions surrounding them are considered to be essential ingredients of the treatment process. In contrast, the systems framework of family therapy views behavioural change as either preceding or occurring without the client necessarily acquiring much insight. Fourth, the analysis and ultimately the interpretation of the transference, which develops between analyst and patient, is the primary treatment tool in psycho-analysis. In analytically oriented casework, the relationship between worker and client is used differently—to offer, for example, a substitutory relationship to a client who has a grossly inadequate psycho-social environment or to provide a corrective emotional experience to overlay an earlier defective one. But in both the analytic and the casework situations, the relationship between *worker and client* is used in a direct way to help to resolve the client's past conflicts and this procedure is the primary motivating force for change. In contrast, the occurrence and use of transference is different in family therapy. The family therapist does not seek to develop a relationship between each individual family member and himself or to make the understanding of transference phenomena a major part of his treatment interventions, although, as in all psychotherapeutic situations, he will need to be aware of the past relationships which each family member transfers on to him and, especially during the later phases of treatment, to help each to test these images against the actuality of his real relationship with him. However, the family therapist's chief concern is the introjected image of the whole family which in turn gets reprojected by each family member on to the real world of his actual family group. It is this system of family transferences which must be his chief focus instead of the client/worker transference of the one-to-one situation. Finally, whilst the psycho-analyst believes that it is possible for an individual to change *in isolation* from his immediate psycho-social environment, the systems theorist views lasting change as essentially involving change within the client's significant others as a total system. Psycho-analysis deals with the symbolic; family therapy with the actual.

Jackson (1967, p. 39) summarises the relationship between psycho-analysis and family theory based on the systems framework as follows: 'Family study, spurred by the accident of conjoint family therapy, has resulted in a body of data that differs significantly from psycho-analytic data. It is not better or worse, it is different.'

## The family myth

Despite these considerable differences, some of the insights of psycho-analysis do, in my view, contribute to GST as a theoretical base for undertaking family therapy; and whilst some schools of family therapy turn their back completely on the psycho-analytic model, most have developed and extended certain key concepts in such a way that they can enrich and harmonise with the general systems framework. Three of these concepts will be examined briefly: family myths; family transference distortions and counter-transference; and the concept of interlocking pathology. As is the case in GST, there is inevitably overlap between some of these concepts.

The concept of family myth has been developed by Ferreira (1963) in the United States, and by Byng-Hall at the Tavistock Clinic, London. Byng-Hall (1973, p. 239) describes the myth as a

pattern of mutually agreed but distorted roles, which family members adopt as a defensive posture and which are not challenged from within the family. . . The myth represents a compromise between family members so that each individual's defences are maintained through the myth. Thus threats to the myth also threaten the individual's defences and changes in individuals threaten the family myth.

The purpose of the family myth is to enable family members and outsiders to remain unaware of 'the avoided theme'. This theme is somewhat analogous to the family 'secret' but usually describes deeply unconscious phenomena. Byng-Hall describes two types of collusion between family members, either of which enables a family myth to be developed: the first is based on the mutual attraction of marital partners to each other derived from their unconscious perception in the other of the repressed, negative, but sought after aspects of their own personality; the second is based on the idealisation of the other and of the relationship between them. These concepts derive from the familiar and earlier work of the Family Discussion Bureau (as it was then called) at the Tavistock Clinic. For example, with regard to the second type of collusion just described, Pincus (1971, p. 14) comments:

> Although there is often a wish to start afresh in marriage and to escape the frustrations or disappointments of unsatisfactory early relationships, a strong unconscious tie to the first love-objects may help to determine the choice of a partner with whom the earlier situation can be compulsively re-enacted.

Byng-Hall, however, develops the Family Discussion Bureau's concepts of marital 'fit' to relate to the whole family system, including the children, and suggests that 'marital collusions which are defending against unresolved child/parent relationships are likely to recruit children into major roles in the defensive system'. Workers at what is now called The Institute of Marital Studies (formerly the Family Discussion Bureau) base their practice largely on their understanding of psycho-analytic theory and the ideas which they and others have developed about marital interaction, rather than on systems theory which encompasses the whole family. They conduct their therapeutic work chiefly via the medium of concurrent or collaborative treatment sessions.[1] Byng-Hall, by using the concept of family myth, has developed these ideas within the framework of a systems approach, and in a way which assists the family therapist in conceptualising the operation of unconscious processes within the family group. This helps us towards a more profound understanding of the concept of wholeness—involving the systemic interrelationship of interpersonal *and* intra-psychic experience. Thus it provides a framework for understanding a seemingly random assignment of irrational roles within the family group. Ackerman (1966a) suggests that the multiplicity of these role assignments can usually be reduced to three main archetypal roles, those of. attacker, healer and victim, the family member being 'selected for his respective role by shared unconscious processes within the group'. Satir (1972) on the other hand suggests the existence of four 'universal patterns of response' or main family roles, those of placater, blamer, computer and distracter. The important aspect of these role assignments is their interrelationship—each person is helped to maintain his own role position within the group, for good or ill, by virtue of the roles exercised by other family members. The family myth has the function of tying together this multiplicity of interlocking role assignments and maintaining them in being. The family therapist needs to gain an understanding both of the roles themselves, and the meaning that they hold within the framework of the family myth.[2]

## Family transference

The concept of family transference has been developed by many family therapists—notably by the group of workers at the Eastern Pennsylvania Psychiatric Institute, led by Boszormenyi-Nagy and by some workers at the Tavistock Clinic, London. The traditional concept of transference is used, but the emphasis is shifted from attaching central importance to the worker/client transference, to viewing intra-familial transference phenomena as of primary importance for the family therapist in understanding and altering family processes (a link is made between the two different emphases, by Ackerman (1959) who reminds us that, 'The root of transference is interaction of individual and family'). The importance of intra-familial transference phenomena is underlined by the family therapy situation itself, and by the therapist's presentation of himself as a real human being. As Barnes (1973, p. 66) remarks, the family therapy situation allows

> The containment of the potential projections . . . within members of the family group. Where the therapist is more active and real, the infantile projections and distortions that occur remain among the family members and can there be pointed out, examined and clarified as they appear in the room during a session.

In attempting to deal with their own unacceptable, frightening and hostile feelings, family members transfer on to each other the 'child' and 'parent' positions which derive from their own past relationships. For example, a mother may transfer on to one of her children the image of her own mother, together with the feelings of persecution she experienced at her mother's hands. She may then view this child as powerfully controlling and 'parental' towards her, which will then obviously affect the way in which she reacts to this child and likewise the way in which the child reacts to her. Husband may transfer on to wife his image of his own mother, as a warm, nurturing dependable person, who could be relied upon to protect him from the consequences of his own actions. If these two sets of transferred feelings occur in the same family, there will be three conflicting mothers within this one family group: the actual real-life mother (who is interacting as a child); the child mother (of mother's transference); and the mother mother (of father's transference). The complexity of the situation is obviously greatly increased when a third generation, in the form of grandparents, is introduced into the treatment situation. Moreover, as some family theorists have pointed out, what is internalised is primarily a sequence of relationships between past significant objects, not the objects or part objects themselves (Laing, 1972, p. 118):

> It is relations not objects that are internalised and the meaning of the relations between events in space and time that counts . . . . Transference consists (among other things) in carrying over one metamorphosis, based on being 'in' and having inside oneself one mode of sociality.

The family therapist is thus confronted with a network of transferred images and relationships, derived from individuals' experiences of significant past relationships and which are frequently (as in the above example) in conflict with each other. His task is to enable the family group to interact in terms of the reality of its current affective relationships, by divesting itself of the 'phantasy family' of members' earlier experiences.

Whilst transference between therapist and individual family member (in the psycho-analytic sense) is of diminished importance in family therapy, the concept of counter-transference becomes correspondingly more central. The family therapist places himself in an emotional system which replicates both his family of origin and his current family situation to varying degrees. He is confronted not only with the real-life members of the family group, but also with a network of transferred relationships and images from *their* past. Both the actual members of the family group and the network of family transferences, can arouse in the family therapist a multiplicity of emotional resonances. Family therapists commonly experience the need to get more 'involved' when working with family groups than when working with individuals. It seems inevitable that the highly charged emotional material which is presented to the therapist when working with families *in vivo,* re-involves him in his own primitive early experiences. It is the very fact that the family therapist carries into the treatment situation an awareness of his own struggles which sharpens his therapeutic potency; yet he must avoid using the families with which he works to re-shape a more adequate and satisfying family milieu for himself. Whitaker *et al.* (1965) warn against both the 'Scylla of over-involvement' and the 'Charybdis of isolation'. Obviously, the caseworker faces a similar dilemma in his work with individuals; but the family therapy situation seems to heighten the therapist's tendency to move too far in either of these two directions. Because of the powerfulness of the family group and the contrasting vulnerability of the single therapist or even the co-therapy pair, the therapist often finds himself thrown back into a child-like posture, experiencing the parents as his own parental figures. This may induce him to make an inappropriate alliance with the identified patient, ostensibly in order to *give* him support, but unconsciously in order to *get* support, in order to withstand the power of the parents. Conversely he may, equally inappropriately, make an alliance with the parents and become 'parental' towards the identified patient—ending up with the tacit agreement to join the parents in their scapegoating game in exchange for their approval. The family therapist must refuse resolutely to become 'sucked in' to the family system whereby he merely dances to the family's tune; yet he must continually develop his ability to use himself freely and flexibly as parent, child, mother, teacher or lover, making and breaking alliances with family members in a manner which continually moves the group, including himself, towards a more mature and satisfying pattern of interaction.

The family therapist must endeavour to 'de-triangulate' himself from his family of origin and from the compulsive effort to resolve his past conflicts via current interpersonal relationships. However, a practical problem confronts the family therapist in his handling of counter-transference phenomena. Whereas the worker involved in the treatment of individuals derives enormous strength from his own personal analysis or other personal psychotherapeutic help, few family therapists receive a comparable experience. In order to work effectively with the family group, a family therapist is obviously greatly assisted by receiving family psychotherapy himself, as a member of either his family of origin or his current family or both. Yet for most of us this is impractical. Nevertheless, as Whitaker *et al.* (1965) point out: 'When he accepts the family as his patient, the therapist begins to expose the immature residuals of his own person.' Hence some personal work needs to be undertaken by the family therapist if he is to be freed sufficiently from his own areas of immaturity to interact effectively in the family group he is treating. In chapters 5 and 8 we will note the help afforded in monitoring one's work by mechanical aids and by the use of co-therapy.

The family therapist will also help himself by consciously directing his affect towards the family group as a whole, reminding himself continually that the whole group is his patient and not any one sub-system of it. His activity within the group does not entail an objective neutrality in the sense of never taking sides, but the family must sense his commitment to their growth as a whole and his ability to be tough, gentle, warm, spontaneous or distant as and when the therapeutic endeavour requires and not simply at the dictates of his own unconscious needs. The family therapy session has been likened to a dance in which family members and therapist(s) weave in and out of each other in a constant inter-play of movement and sound (Watermann, 1971). The therapist must endeavour to use steps which will assist the family in their struggle to choreograph a new dance sequence.

## Interlocking pathology

Our third concept, derived from psycho-analytic theory is that of interlocking pathology. Well before therapists began treating family groups in their hospitals and agencies, many workers had noted the interrelated nature of much symptomatology. In chapter 1, reference was made to the work of Johnson and Szurek who noted the way in which children seemed sometimes to act out their parents' forbidden impulses and family therapy received much of its impetus from the disquieting observations of analysts and caseworkers who noticed that, sometimes, when their patient improved, his marriage broke up. In the previous chapter, we looked at symptoms as a means of displaced communication within the family system. At this point, we will note briefly the way in which family therapists working from a psycho-analytic standpoint have come to view symptomatology within the economy of the family group. Framo (1970, p. 127) writes: 'Departing from the conventional, simplistic view of symptoms as intra-psychic entities and as stemming from a central illness' it is the author's view that 'symptoms are formed, selected, faked, exchanged, maintained and reduced as a function of the relationship context in which they are naturally embedded.'

The concept of interlocking pathology covers several different aspects concerning the reciprocal and interrelated nature of unconscious processes within the family group. Such ideas have been variously described as the trading of dissociations (Wynne, 1965); mutual secondary gains (Framo, 1970); the unconscious transmission of feelings (Jordan, 1970); and the exchange of symptoms. 'The essential thesis behind the transpersonal view of psychopathology is that people really do have an effect upon one another when they are in close relationships, a telling effect, which is more than the resultant of two interacting intra-psychic systems', comments Framo (1965). The way in which family members get other family members to carry certain feelings on their behalf is a more complicated process than the psycho-analytic concept of projection. Yet Freud himself discussed (though did not develop) the idea of the unconscious transmission of feelings as early as 1915 in his paper 'The unconscious': 'It is very remarkable that the unconscious of one human being can react upon that of another, without the conscious being implicated at all.' But it was only gradually that this phenomenon came to be recognised in psychotherapeutic practice, and the full import of the idea only became apparent after conjoint family and marital work began to be practised. Thus the symptom bearer is seen as undertaking a specific emotional task for one or more other members of the family group. For example: a widowed mother and her two sons aged 12 and 14 years were seen in conjoint family interviews over a period of a year. The symptom was presented by David, the 14 year old, who was enuretic and who had recurrent, horrifying nightmares revolving around the theme of death. He was also preoccupied with a morbid interest in churchyards and funerals and would not leave his mother either to go to school or to mix with friends of his own age. During the course of treatment, it materialised that mother was suffering from a severely inhibited grief reaction—she had barely cried for or spoken about her husband since his death ten years earlier. Her sons had grown up in this atmosphere of total restraint which ultimately found its outlet through David's compensatory preoccupation with death, combined with his enuretic 'weeping'. When mother began to mourn for her husband and to talk about her loneliness, David's nightmares and morbid waking interest in death ceased; he began to make friends and go to school, and his enuresis improved. In this family, David expressed his mother's grief symbolically on her behalf. One could describe this process in terms of an exchange of symptoms; or an unconscious transmission of feelings whereby mother required her son to carry her unexpressed grief in a symbolic manner; or one could view the process in terms of the mutual secondary gains derived by mother (who did not have to face the pain of her grief) and David (who did not have to face the challenge of leaving his mother's side or mixing with his peers). Whichever concept is utilised, the family therapist is witnessing and using a transactional phenomenon in terms of the family's system of unconscious processes.

Sometimes the emotional 'lightning' within the family group is only 'earthed' when an outsider such as a family therapist is introduced. For example: a family was referred for treatment consisting of mother and her two children, together with her common law husband, with whom she had cohabited for the past two years. I had read the referral letter carefully, in which it was stated that there were two children; and I had spoken to mother over the telephone, to check that the appointment was convenient. During this telephone conversation, I again established that there were only two children. However, for the first interview I placed chairs for the adults and for *three* children. As soon as I commented on my mistake, mother broke down, crying that although she had never told anyone before, she longed for a child of this, her present relationship. Without such a child, she felt that the family that she and her boyfriend were trying to create was incomplete. Somehow it seemed that mother had transmitted her acutely painful feelings concerning this missing child to me even though the communication was entirely unconscious, both in its expression from mother and in its response from me.

In a recent article, Wertheim (1973) attempts a comparative overview of the main theoretical positions currently held by family therapists. She compares three propositions: SI (Supra-Individual); SII (Supra-Individual/Individual); and SIISF (Supra-Individual/Individual/Supra-Family). The SI position describes that of the family therapist working from the general systems theory. The SII position describes that of the family therapist who, whilst working within the systems framework, utilises concepts from individual treatment modalities—as described in this chapter. The SIISF position extends the family therapist's area of interest and concern to include the interface between family and community in addition to the interface between family member and family group and is employed by those who practise network therapy and multiple family therapy. The two latter positions—SII and SIISF—extend and refine the systems view of family therapy focused within the SI position. The SII position helps to answer the criticism that family therapy loses the individual in its attention to the group (Pearson, 1974); on the other hand, the SIISF position meets the criticism that family therapy loses the outside community—the family's supra-system—in its focus on a single family unit (Busfield, 1974). None of these three positions need be mutually exclusive; and the fact that a more comprehensive description of family therapy theory is being attempted, reflects the greater degree of sophistication which the method has now achieved.

## Notes

1 Personal communication (1974). I am indebted to Mrs Clemency Chapman of the Institute of Marital Studies for providing me with the results of a recent survey of the current practice at the IMS. According to this survey, 68 per cent of cases are treated other than by conjoint marital therapy.
2 A selection of family myths frequently found by family therapists is given by Glick and Hessler (1974), chapter 3. Obviously there are strong cultural connotations involved in both the building up of the myth by the family and in its discernment and evaluation by the therapist.

# Chapter four

# Engaging the family in treatment

. . . rather bear those ills we have
Than fly to others that we know not of.

*Hamlet,* Act 3, Scene 1

Engagement is a process beginning with the therapist's very first contact with the family. It ends when therapist and family have entered into a working relationship which is firm enough to enable both to withstand the painfulness of change, but flexible enough to make continued change possible. The process may take a few minutes or many months. In any event, the success with which the therapist accomplishes this initial phase, determines in large measure the outcome of treatment. Whilst the engagement process necessarily differs with every family and every family therapist, there are a number of aspects to which all family therapists need to address themselves, with each new family.

## Initial contact

The first contact with the family therapist will come either directly from a member of the family, or via a third party, the referrer. In the first instance, the family member may telephone, write or present himself or herself in person at the office. Whoever has the first contact with this family member influences the engagement process. Thus, the person on the telephone switchboard, the receptionist who opens the door or the intake worker who sits at her desk—all influence the possible future course of treatment in a significant way. When the family is referred by another agency, the family therapist's first task is to engage in some meaningful exchange with the referrer. Is he referring the family because of the family's needs or because of his own—or both? Does he feel ambivalent about

35

family therapy, and if so has he communicated this ambivalence to the family? Is he covertly hostile? If so, has he waited to refer the family until the situation has deteriorated into unmitigated chaos, leaving the family therapist able only to pick up a few pieces? On the other hand, the referrer, while consciously wishing to refer the family, may feel, on another level, reluctant to part with them, and place various obstacles in the therapist's way. All these eventualities are possible! Whatever the situation, it is essential for the family therapist to engage in *direct contact with the family as soon as possible*. Normally, he will need to write to the family, inviting them to come to a first interview, or arranging to visit them in their home for this first meeting. In this letter, it is essential that the therapist reminds himself that the *whole family* is his client, and that he must therefore address the letter to each person who seems to be an active part of the family system. At this stage, the therapist will necessarily be relying on the referrer or family member who made initial contact, to help him to judge to whom he should be writing. A useful rule of thumb is to invite everyone who comprises the household. After the first meeting, it may become obvious that other people not actually living in the house should be included, as we will note later on. The choice of venue also has to be made. On the whole, there is much to be said for arranging the first session on territory other than the family's own home, if this is at all possible. The family may feel that it has been given a more open choice as to whether or not to answer the therapist's invitation to engage in the treatment process. The therapist, for his part, may feel that family members, by coming out of their home, have 'voted with their feet' for his involvement in their difficulties. The obvious choice of venue is the therapist's office, if his agency supplies him with one which is suitable. Otherwise, a room in another agency, or part of the agency, such as a sitting room in a day centre, can be used and is often preferable to making the first session a home visit. Whatever the choice, the therapist should make it clear in his letter that he will want to see the whole family and that this meeting will, hopefully, be the beginning of a working contract with them.

### The first interview

The first interview in family therapy involves a unique situation. By the time the family members arrive, they have been able to cope sufficiently with the anxiety engendered by the referrer's discussion with them, and by the therapist's letter of invitation, to make a commitment to a family therapist for at least one session or part of a session. This has involved some recognition of pain or problems existing within the family (probably perceived as being located in one member) and some ability to engage in an activity expressly demanding a co-operative effort. However, despite verbal protestations to the contrary, the family's attitude towards change will be almost wholly negative, since symptomatology is the means whereby the family's homeostasis is maintained. The family's interaction during this first encounter with the therapist, will, to a greater or lesser extent, be directed towards meeting its unconscious need to overthrow the therapist's efforts to act as a therapist. 'The family's task is to try to dismiss us: our task as therapists is to refuse to be dismissed', comments Kempler (1975). Inevitably, therefore, there has to be some kind of struggle between the family and the therapist commencing at the outset of the first interview, which, if successfully negotiated, will result in the formation of a new system made up of family group + family therapist. This system will display the properties of a true system—but each of the two major sub-systems within it must retain the properties which are unique to each. *The family* is responsible for bringing itself into treatment and for struggling, with the help of the therapist, to clarify the way in which it sees its problems and in defining what it wants to change. In other words, the family must define the treatment goals. *The therapist's* initial task is to establish himself as therapist—in charge of the therapeutic process. This means that he has to set boundaries, and draw up a contract for the continuing relationship in treatment of both parts of this new system. Some family therapists, for example Charles Fulweiler, start the first session by giving the family some description of how he views the therapeutic process (1967); others prefer to demonstrate the nature of the process by starting to work straight away, feeding back to the family the interactional patterns as they emerge. The *family* has been able to produce sufficient motivation to come to the first interview—but it is the therapist's interventions during the first session which enable the family to come again. This first session needs, therefore, to be a therapeutic, working encounter—a real meeting of persons, so that the family goes away feeling that change is possible, without the total destruction of its present system.

## The place of history

In family therapy, therefore, the first session is never an administrative, history-taking affair. Nor does the family therapist come to his first meeting with the family armed with an extensive case-history from the previous worker. In fact, coming to the first session with as little information about the family as possible is a very useful practice for the therapist to adopt. It enables him to begin to sensitise himself to the uniqueness of the newly formed system of which he finds himself a part.

The family therapist does not need to collect a 'history' before he can proceed to offer treatment; he has before him the most significant gestalt of all; the current interactions, verbal and non-verbal, of family members in the here and now of the therapy session will reveal the family's areas of pain and strength. This is not to say that most family therapists adopt a totally a-historical approach; it is often useful, especially during the engagement phase, when the family's anxiety level is high, to dip into one or more family member's 'process of becoming', in order temporarily to reduce the current tension of the session. To look for a similar experience to that of a scapegoated family member in another member's past can, for example, shift the focus of pain and reduce anxiety without allowing the family to escape into flight from the problem. This type of procedure can often produce some feeling of empathy within another member of the family for the currently identified patient's position. The exploration of historical material can build up the family's feeling of identity—for example, an acting-out adolescent can get an entirely new view of his role in the family by listening to his parents recall some of their adolescent experiences in relation to *their* parents. History is always for the *family* rather than for the therapist; and its exploration needs to be in dynamic relationship to the current interactional difficulties which the family is experiencing. In order to make historical exploration an involving experience for the whole family, it is helpful to use a blackboard or large sheet of paper and to construct a genogram or genealogy of the family— writing up names, and significant dates and setting out past relationships in the diagrammatic form of a genealogical table. This conversion of the verbal into the visual is a creative way of enlisting the attention and interest of children, in material which may well be completely new to them—and which may become the starting point from which to develop new empathic dialogue across the genera-tional boundaries. It is also a great help in enabling the therapist to retain an enormous amount of new data in some sort of orderly sequence. If a genogram has been started in the first session, it should be kept and be available if the family in future sessions wishes to return to develop or retrieve further memories from their past. It cannot be emphasised too much that this type of historical exploration needs to be undertaken from within the context of the current affective climate of the session; its purpose is always to catalyse the present not to seek for 'causes' in the past. The technique has a limited place for most family therapists and needs to be used with great care in order to avoid a flight from the present by either family or therapist.

## Assessment

Treatment of the family group starts from the first moments of the first interview. The therapist cannot afford to wait until he has clarified and mentally compartmentalised what seems to him to be going on. He takes each fragment of the picture and reflects upon it with the family as it is happening. For example, the first comment made by the family about how things are with them is often the way they choose to sit in the room. It is always useful if the therapist lets the family make this choice, and to take special note of the place the family leave for him. If, for example, they leave a place for him in the middle of their group, where he has difficulty in seeing the whole group at a glance, he might conclude that, on one level, the family wishes to reduce his potency and potential for helping. If this is how the therapist senses his position, he would make a powerful therapeutic intervention by asking a family member to change places with him—thus confronting the family's power to render him impotent in a significant non-verbal way. Again, in another situation, father and the children may sit closely together, with mother a little distance apart, next to the male therapist. It might take many sessions to get a full understanding of what that arrangement means, by which time the moment has long since passed and the therapist has got himself trapped into the stance of some distant commentator. Instead, the family therapist might say: 'You seem to be a bit outside the family, Mother' or (to mother) 'It's nice to have you sitting close', or (to father and children) 'You three look as though you enjoy each other's company'. Each of these comments have both a diagnostic *and* a therapeutic flavour and illustrate the way in which diagnosis and treatment are concurrent not consecutive activities in family therapy. There are many other comments which might be made, depending on the unique affective climate of those first few minutes of the session. Looking at these three interventions, the first is probably the most challenging and the third is likely to be therapeutically most useful in his primary task of healing and change. Thus, while from the purely *diagnostic* point of view each comment has some value, and addresses itself to different aspects of the family + family therapist group, the therapist must give equal importance and attention, from the very first moment, to the sensitivity of his *therapeutic* interventions.

Whilst the family therapist does not try to separate diagnosis and treatment there is a sense in which he needs to make particular use of the first one or two meetings with the family to work towards helping it to formulate some treatment goals and to construct a contract for future work. The therapist needs to appraise, with the family, its communication patterns, its internal alliances, the roles

39

which different family members carry and also the way in which the system affects him as therapist. What position does the family ask him to fill in their system? Does he, as in the above example, experience the wife's need of him as a surrogate husband, even while father may be stating that they have a very happy marriage? He needs to consider the family in terms of its systemic properties of 'openness' and 'closedness' and arrive at some impression of whether it seems to be either enmeshed or disorganised. Moreover, the therapist needs to determine the degree of homeostasis which is operating within the system. Is one individual required to act as a homeostatic regulator? If so, is it the identified patient, or another family member, or is this the role which he, the therapist, is being called upon to play? How far does the family system's inter-relation with its supra-system affect its dysfunctional pattern of interaction? Which sub-speciality of family therapy is most appropriately employed in this case?

Here, we should note that the family therapist relies much more heavily on the *non-verbal process* of the session than on its *verbal content* to supply him with diagnostic clues. At what point in the parents' description of their problems do the small children create a diversion? What is happening in another part of the family when the baby starts to cry? Does the family dog put his nose instinctively into the lap of the person in most pain—even though that person always wears a defensive smile? When small children are playing in the session, it is always worth pausing to review the sort of messages they are giving about the family through the non-verbal medium of their play material. For example, while the parents are assuring the therapist that theirs would be an idyllically happy family if it were not for Johnnie's bed-wetting, Johnnie may be drawing a picture of a house in a thunderstorm. When working with a single mother and her 8 year old daughter, the therapists noticed that while mother was denying that her daughter might be interested in her father, the little girl was making 'families' out of plasticine, consisting of mothers and babies only. When the male therapist picked up some plasticine and made a family, consisting of mother, baby and father, the little girl shouted: 'Baby is dead. It is sad and crying because she is not sleeping with Mum'—followed after a short pause by 'If Daddy comes back I would be taken away.' The family therapist needs to be constantly 'tuned in' to discrepancies between verbal content and non-verbal process, remembering that it is a person's non-verbal expressions of himself and his place in the family system, that are the least censored and inhibited. The therapist's diagnostic task is to try to translate the seemingly random non-verbal activities of individuals into a pattern which is meaningful in terms of the whole system.

## Establishing the ground rules

The therapist starts establishing various important 'ground rules' of family therapy from the beginning of the first session. The fact that they have been invited to come as a family group, at once establishes the basic and most fundamental premise of family therapy. The therapist needs to go on conveying the message that it is the group as a whole that interests him and that he will not simply be treating an individual in the presence of his family. He will need to avoid being trapped by 'secret' information given by one family member about another, either over the telephone between sessions, or when a family member hangs back after the rest have gone, in order to convey to the therapist what he 'could not possibly say in front of the others'. It is important to let the family know early on that, whilst hopefully everyone (including the therapist) will become able to say what they wish to each other during the sessions, there may be things which an individual does not feel able to share with the whole group straight away. For his part, the therapist must help the family to understand that whatever a family member shares with *him* he will consider to be the property of the whole group and share it with them. It is far better for the therapist to remain 'in the dark' than to become privy to some highly charged private information about an individual which he cannot use, and which thus seriously hampers his spontaneity and freedom of movement in the sessions.

It is important to try to establish an atmosphere of openness and intimacy. The best way to do this is for the therapist to try to model it for the family—by, for example, sharing his feelings of nervousness, bewilderment or confusion as he sits down with them. He may also choose to introduce himself by his first name, suggesting that first names be used in the sessions as a way of encouraging everyone to work towards a greater degree of openness, sharing and intimacy during their meetings together. With some families, and in some agency situations, such a procedure undertaken early in the first session would be premature, or remain inappropriate throughout treatment; the important point to try to establish is this culture of openness, and to use whatever seems comfortable and natural to the family and therapist in trying to achieve this atmosphere. It is clearly a great help if the therapist can use a room which is comfortably and informally furnished. If it is only possible to use a formal room, then the desk should be pushed back, and a circle of chairs arranged, using as far as possible, chairs of similar heights and sizes.

It is important for the therapist to establish a meaningful relationship with each member of the group, in a way which is appropriate to the age, sex and emotional needs of each individual. Each member of the group must feel the therapist's interest and concern for himself or herself, so that he can begin to feel, however unclearly, that there may be something to be gained by him personally, if he comes to the sessions. The first and second sessions are characterised by the therapist's efforts to join with the family to form the new group of family + therapist. In so far as this union is an 'arranged marriage' via a referrer, more effort and skill is required on the therapist's part in successfully negotiating this union, and in emerging from the second session having formulated a working contract with the family.

## Shifting the focus to the family group

Families present themselves for treatment either symptomatically in terms of an *individual* in trouble, or interactionally in terms of difficulties within a *relationship*—between marital partners or parent and child, for example. Most usually, the therapist is presented with the first alternative, where the family views the source of all its difficulties as lying within one of its members. In chapters 2 and 3, we noted some of the complex issues surrounding the family's need for an identified patient. At the outset of treatment the family and the therapist meet with widely disparate views of both how the family's trouble is caused and the way in which the difficulties might be alleviated. The family will often feel that its distress would be relieved if the symptomatic individual is removed or magically changed. The therapist will view the individual's symptomatology as calling attention to fundamental areas of dysfunction within the family's internal relationships. His concern is with the politics of the family, not the pathology of the individual. At this juncture, the family and the therapist are systems in collision. The therapist has to steer the difficult middle course between, on the one hand, collusion with the family and consequent loss of therapeutic leverage and, on the other, an insistence on premature change within the family system, bringing consequent loss of the family. It is fruitless for the therapist to ignore a parent's cry for help regarding his son's stealing, or to maintain that 'this is not the problem in the family'. It manifestly *is* the problem at the commencement of treatment. On the other hand, to allow the family to feel that the therapist unreservedly shares its view of the stealing, would reinforce the system's scapegoating mechanism and alienate the identified patient.

The handling of the identified patient poses the family therapist with special problems from the outset of treatment. It is often a tremendous relief for this individual if the therapist is able to convey the message that he does not share the family's view of his place in their system and it is usually vital to try to convey this message during the first session. It is often useful for the therapist to sit next to the identified patient; sometimes the non-verbal support that can be given by this physical proximity enables this individual to function a little more freely during the session. The fact that this person has become symptomatic, indicates that he is predisposed by his own psychodynamic make-up and emotional needs towards fulfilling the role of trouble shooter. He is often extremely sensitive to the underlying emotional needs of others and can thus be of assistance to the therapist in eliciting a fuller view of the family's difficulties. He is often the therapist's point of entry into the family system. When asking each family member how they see the trouble in the family, the identified patient will often come forward with a radically different view from that of other family members—sometimes to their great surprise. In this situation, the identified patient feels strengthened by the neutral, protective, caring presence of the therapist, and the family is often able to begin to tackle their problems from the new starting point offered by the identified patient, for the first time. At this stage, some sort of bargaining takes place between the therapist and the identified patient—the identified patient providing the therapist with his entry point into the family system in return for the protection he experiences from the therapist. Although this can offer a useful alliance at first, the therapist needs to be wary of placing too much reliance on this 'marriage'; for the identified patient is just as likely to call the family out of treatment at a later stage when further layers of the onion have been removed, and he has begun to realise that change and growth is required of him also.

## Constructing a contract

By the end of the second session it is hopefully possible to formulate a working contract with the family. This contract will place some boundaries around the ongoing relationship between the family and the therapist. A contract may be defined as (Goldstein, 1973, p. 137):

> the organised set of explicitly or tacitly understood ways in which the interactors in a system agree to carry on their business . . . what is involved is not only an assumption of responsibility for the roles and tasks required to achieve a desired end but also a warrant to maintain and sustain the change system.

This contract represents an important step in creating a therapeutic system out of the two sub-systems of family + family therapist and, to be effective it must cover the following areas. First, an attempt at defining treatment goals must be made and the contract between family and family therapist needs to be made concrete around some specific aims and purposes. The goals which the therapeutic system of family + family therapist sets for itself will be limited by the potential for growth inherent within each particular system. Since change, however small or great, will inevitably encompass the whole therapeutic system during the course of its existence, goals need to emerge, as far as possible, out of the process of the system itself. The therapeutic system will need to address itself to defining different levels and priorities in selecting its goals. Goldstein (1973) has suggested five different levels on which goals can be categorised: concrete; current reality; structural; foresight and vitalistic goals. The family therapy contract can embrace all or any of these levels, but it will always include structural goals, by which the system itself is modified, developed and changed. These initially defined goals must be capable of continual modification and development throughout the course of treatment and will encompass both optimal and interim objectives at different stages of the treatment process.

Second, the therapist must formulate some answer to the basic but complex question—'Who constitutes the family in this particular case?' In other words, what is the operative family system with which work must be undertaken? Modifications will take place later, but during this engagement phase, it is essential that the therapist makes an initial decision as to which family members should come to the sessions. During the first two sessions, it may have become apparent that a grandparent living with the family is vitally involved in the family's difficulties and is therefore needed. In a marital situation, husband may be trying to work through a triangular relationship involving his wife and his girl friend. The triangular system thus formed would probably be the operative family system which the therapist would need in treatment. It may be that during the first two sessions, a child that was signalling the family's distress by school refusal has felt sufficiently re-assured that the underlying difficulties in his parents' marriage can be helped, for him to return to school. This sort of dramatic abatement of the symptom is not unusual, and often allows the therapist to drop the identified patient from the sessions altogether—continuing work with the marital pair. Alternatively, it may seem important to work with the families of origin of each of the marital pair—if they are available—and move to the current family situation later on in the treatment process. In every situation, the composition of the therapy group is a treatment decision, and as such, is the responsibility of the therapist, not the family. Refusing to bring an essential component of the family system to the sessions is a standard means of resistance on the part of the family and poses the therapist with a serious challenge, at any stage in the treatment process. However, if the family refuses to bring essential members to the sessions at the outset, the outcome of treatment is almost certain to be unsuccessful. Thus, an essential task during this engagement phase is to enable the family to bring the operative system, or the minimum sufficient network, as Skynner (1971) has described it, into treatment.

Third, the contract should include a decision regarding venue. Again, this is a treatment decision and it should be made by the therapist in accordance with the emotional needs of the family. If the symptomatic family member is agoraphobic, it might be useful to commence sessions in the family's home, and work towards eventually holding them in the office. If there is the possibility of using audio and video recordings or a one-way observation screen, and if these aids are judged to be useful in working with a particular case, this would be an indication for deciding to hold the sessions in the office. Whatever the decision, it is important that the therapist maintains the option to be flexible, since it is usually helpful to make a change in the venue for at least one session during the course of treatment. For example, with a family who customarily come to the office, the therapist might wish to arrange a home visit to facilitate the transfer of the work to the home setting. On the other hand, with a family whom the therapist usually meets at home, a session held in the office would make the use of audio-visual aids possible for this one occasion.

Finally, the contract may embrace some decision regarding the length, frequency and number of sessions. Some family therapists prefer to work in short intensive periods of perhaps three months, then recess the family, and formulate a new working contract with them after a break of two or three months. This combines the advantages of brief intervention with those of follow up and a further period of work. Other therapists think in terms of longer periods of work from the outset of treatment, and do not normally decide on a fixed number of sessions during the engagement phase.

## The therapist's use of himself

The way in which the therapist uses his own personality during the course of treatment is a distinctive feature of family therapy. As noted in chapter 3, the family therapist's primary focus is the real world of the family's current relationships. His use and handling of transference phenomena tend to be in terms of the family's internal projections from one family member to another, rather than, as in the individual casework relationship, in terms of the client's transference to the therapist. Whilst part of the caseworker's task is to enable the client to project internal images onto him, the family therapist seeks to use the whole of his psychodynamic make-up in a flexible, involved manner and to enter into the family system as a human being rather than as a professional person. This involves taking on the dual role of participant and observer *vis-à-vis* the family system, moving in and out of these two roles in accordance with the therapeutic needs of the family. It is important that the therapist demonstrates to the family, early on in the engagement process, that he will sometimes be an active participant, and sometimes an observer of family processes. Otherwise, it may be difficult for him later on, to move from one position to the other as the need arises. To establish his role as an observer during the first session, he may, for example, ask family members to talk to *each other* about their difficulties, not to the therapist. If there is a one way viewing screen in the room, he might go behind the screen and watch the family for a while, returning to feed back to them his observations of their interaction. To establish himself as a participant, he might comment: 'I'm beginning to feel pretty anxious at the moment, looking at Mum's and Dad's angry faces. I wonder whether your feelings, Johnnie, are at all the same?' A simple empathic intervention of this kind establishes the therapist's intention to use himself as a 'feeling barometer' early in the therapeutic process and helps to declare himself and the way he intends to work openly for the family to experience.

The dysfunctional family challenges, by its frozen immobility, the therapist's flexible and mobile use of himself. The therapist's work is often greatly accelerated by the extent to which he can encourage emotional mobility by the use of physical mobility in the sessions. Thus, it is useful if the therapist can feel free enough to move his physical position in the group, to touch family members, to move in and out of the room, if a one way screen is available—and to encourage a similar mobility within the family. More important still, the therapist needs to free himself to be *emotionally* mobile within the family—able to use the maternal, nurturing parts of his personality as well as the tougher, controlling parts appropriately. This kind of mobility can, like every other technique, be used as a defence against pain as well as a challenge to growth. Growth springs from silence and acceptance as well as from movement and change: from stillness as well as from activity. The therapist's responsibility is to make possible a freedom of choice in terms of therapeutic technique and therefore in terms of therapeutic outcome for the family.

# Chapter five

# The treatment process

O wad some Power
the giftie gie us
To see oursels as
ithers see us!
          Robert Burns

Within the general framework of systems theory, as outlined in chapter 2, family therapists have been essentially pragmatic in their approach to the treatment of psycho-social dysfunction. Partly due to the early application of family therapy to the intractable problems of chronic schizophrenia, when almost anything seemed worth trying, the method has been characterised from the beginning by a preparedness to experiment. This spirit of eclecticism has remained and has contributed to a sense of adventure and continual discovery. Family therapy's concern is with the solution of problems rather than with the strict adherence to theoretical dogma. As a result, its practitioners have been prepared to draw for assistance upon treatment approaches differing as widely as psycho-analysis and encounter group work; behaviour modification and psycho-drama, to the extent to which these approaches have seemed compatible with the theory of general systems. The next three chapters will examine a variety of treatment techniques derived from different sources. Obviously different therapists will find some of these congenial, whilst others will appear less useful or even distasteful.

  The manner in which therapists select and build up a repertoire of intervention techniques is interesting in itself. In practice, the choice and use of a particular technique depends more upon that elusive quality we call 'style', than it does upon the particular theoretical orientation of the therapist.[1] The individual style of the family therapist is the end-product of all those influences on his personal

47

and professional life which go to make up the unique manner in which he practises his art. His personality, his value system and his cultural background influence a therapist's style of working more significantly than the exact theoretical framework on which he draws; and although attempts have been made to link therapeutic style with theoretical orientation these seem to me to be unconvincing.

The most thoroughgoing description and comparison of different styles of work by Beels and Ferber (1969) distinguishes two types of family therapists: 'the reactors' and 'the conductors'. The reactors take a more passive role in the treatment process, emphasising the need to push the family back upon its own resources and encouraging it to retain responsibility for its own change and growth. These therapists emphasise the use of family members' free associations—both through their verbal comments and their non-verbal activities within the session. The reactive therapist is more likely to comment upon the family's interaction in such a way as to encourage change rather than to initiate change directly himself. Verbal techniques, such as interpretation, are used somewhat more freely and the course of treatment is usually more prolonged. In contrast, the conductors feel comfortable in initiating change and in challenging growth. They may be directive and demanding in their relationship to the family and make use of tasks in encouraging the family towards achieving its treatment goal. They emphasise the use of less verbal techniques and often engage in short-term treatment. Haley (1962) too, provides an amusing yet thought-provoking description of the varying styles adopted by family therapists. There is the 'Stone Wall School' in which the family has to struggle to find a meeting ground with the uncompromisingly 'differentiated' therapist. There is the 'Dignified School' where family members find that the therapist gives weight and acceptance to all the differing and conflicting opinions within the group and yet somehow manages to propel the family towards a novel solution without anyone being quite aware of what has happened. Then there is the 'Brotherly Love School' in which the therapists engulf the family with positive feelings and re-interpret their every destructive comment in a constructive manner. The 'Chuck It and Run School' describes those therapists who emphasise the family's inherent capacity to change itself, which they underline by disappearing as often as possible behind a one-way viewing screen, emerging only to make suggestions when things appear to be going wrong. Haley caricatures various other schools of family therapy, each describing a particular style of work. In this chapter, consideration will be given to some *basic* techniques utilised by therapists of different working styles and some attention will be devoted to particular problems arising at different stages of the treatment process.

**Coupling techniques**

Having successfully engaged the family in treatment, the therapist next has to stay 'coupled' with the family and to enable family members to continue coming to the sessions, despite the inevitable pain and anxiety. Whilst the therapist's overall objective is to help the family to change its dysfunctional patterns of interaction, the change-producing techniques which he adopts must always be sensitively tempered with interventions designed to lower the stress and anxiety involved in change. This procedure echoes the way in which the caseworker blends sustaining techniques with those designed to increase insight. Vital as coupling techniques are in family therapy they have received little attention in the literature. The exception is some work undertaken by Minuchin (1974a), in which he analyses these interventions with great clarity, identifying three separate procedures: maintenance; tracking; and mimesis. Each enables the therapist to undertake the essential function of staying 'coupled' with the family for the period of time necessary for change to take place.

'*Maintenance*' involves supporting the *structure* of the family group in terms of its coalitions and alliances at the point when these are being threatened by the therapist's efforts to bring about change. For example: whilst the treatment goal in working with a marital pair may be to enable the husband to share in decision-making and to assert some of his own needs more forcefully, his wife may need the therapist's strong support whilst she is struggling to relinquish her monopoly over this side of their married life. The therapist may seem to 'collude' in maintaining the '*status quo*' at the point when the wife's anxiety rises beyond the level at which she could continue coming to the sessions. When her anxiety has subsided through the therapist's supportive intervention, movement and change may be possible once again.

'*Tracking*' is described by Minuchin as (1974a):

a method of adopting the *content* of family communications. . . . In tracking, the therapist does not challenge the family. It is a method which has its roots in hypnotic suggestion, in which the patient is never confronted. If the patient refuses a suggestion, the hypnotist accepts his refusal but manipulates the situation so that the refusal is a form of obeying the hypnotist's command (italics mine).

For example: a family consisting of step-father, John, and mother, Mary (who are unmarried) and two children, a boy aged 11, Steven, and a girl aged 9, Jane, had been in treatment for six weeks, because of the boy's behaviour problems, expressed both at home and at school. John and Mary's relationship was potentially a fruitful one and the children had welcomed John into the family as their father. The sessions focused around the family's difficulty in determining its own boundary in relation to neighbours, extended family and the wider community (including the school), for it soon became clear that Steven's difficulties were reactive to the uncertain continuity of the family group. John and Mary lacked confidence in their relationship *vis-à-vis* the outside world. They felt angry and undermined by the intrusion of other people into their family life— neighbours critical of their co-habitation; relatives intrusive with their advice on how to bring up the children; and the school, questioning and critical about the differences in surname between children and parents. Yet neither parent felt confident in *excluding* friends or relatives from their family life. On the other hand, Mary was ambivalent about the extent to which she was prepared to *include* John in bringing up the children or how far she would allow him to discipline them. Early treatment goals were established by which John would replace Mary's parents as the final authority in matters concerning the children's upbringing; and the family would struggle with the problem of how to integrate David, Mary's husband, into their emotional system. Whilst John and Mary agreed that they both wanted to exclude David, and prevent his frequent, unscheduled visits, the children felt more ambivalent and on the whole seemed to want to see their father from time to time. The session which followed the children's first expression of this ambivalence commenced with Mary and John announcing that they had decided to take a firm stand and prevent the children's father visiting in the future. During the previous week they had consulted a solicitor and found that they could legally take this step under certain conditions. They had also made detailed enquiries about how to deal with some of the legal road blocks standing in the way of John's divorce and consequently of their marriage. As a result, they did not want to continue with the sessions, as they 'knew that I would not approve'. Despite this, they intended to go through with their plan, as they felt that it was the only way in which John would be able to become a real part of the family and feel confident enough to act as father towards the children. Although from the point of view of the children's long-term emotional needs and wishes, John and Mary's total ban on their father's visits seemed a backward step, nevertheless it demonstrated a dramatic change in the ability of this couple to act decisively and confidently as the leaders of the family group, instead of being influenced, controlled and directed by well-meaning outsiders. Their reaction to me was, I felt, a way of testing out their capacity to take charge of their situation *vis-à-vis* an outsider. I did not therefore challenge their decision or in any way intervene to support the children who were expressing objections. To challenge the parents would be to lose the family from treatment just at a time when their action was in itself a major step towards the overall treatment objective. My interventions were therefore directed towards reinforcing the positive step they had been able to take in cementing John more firmly into the family and in asserting their ability to survive and continue as a group. The family did not terminate treatment prematurely and Steven's behaviour difficulties began to improve markedly from this point onwards. In this instance the therapist 'tracked' the *content* of the family's interactions, becoming swept 'off course' along with the children. Nevertheless, the family continued to be propelled towards their overall treatment goals and as a result Steven's symptomatology abated.

*Mimesis* denotes the coupling technique by which the family's style, affect, culture and mood are incorporated by the therapist into his own interactions with family members. It signifies the way in which the therapist accommodates himself to the family's *affective process*. It involves an ever-responsive sensitivity on the therapist's part to the changing mood and affect of the group from session to session, as well as an ability to respond appropriately to the wide differences in culture, language and socio-economic customs which will characterise each family. The therapist's manner and response must necessarily be different when working with an indigenous West Indian family than when working with an immigrant Pakistani family. It must be different when working with a poor, working-class family from a slum clearance area, than when working with a middle-class family from a suburban estate. Because the family therapist seeks to join the family system as a participant, as well as to engage with it as an observer of its processes, there is perhaps an even greater need than in casework for the worker to be able to employ the family's own modes of expression and to adopt its cultural norms. He does not do this in an artificial, self-conscious manner, but intuitively and spontaneously as a natural means of seeking the privilege of belonging to them as therapist. Coupling operations can therefore be directed towards the *structure, content* or *affective process* within the family group. They are required throughout the course of treatment, whenever stress and anxiety go beyond the level of tolerance and threaten to close family members' defences or remove them from treatment altogether. The use of coupling techniques is far removed from the unconscious collusion of the therapist who finds himself hopelessly manipulated and out-manoeuvred by the family, with the treatment goals receding further and further into the distance. On the contrary, these techniques, designed to maintain the family in treatment, allow family and therapist to continue their relationship long enough for the treatment goals to be achieved. In practice, coupling involves a preparedness to discuss problems, admit mistakes, and be emotionally available to family members as and when the need arises within the sessions.


## Defined problem-solving

The family therapy session is a slice of real life. It provides the therapist with a re-enactment of the ongoing patterns of behaviour which occur between family members during the times when he is not with them. The idea of taking hold of small pieces of interaction as they are offered by the family, springs from the belief that the 'manipulation of the present is the tool for changing the present and the future' (Minuchin, 1974a). The family therapist does not meet the family with any fixed agenda, but tries to work towards resolving small, symbolic conflicts as they are manifested within the session. This may take the form of examining and using the anxiety which is aroused by the session itself, as in the following example. In this extract, the therapists were meeting the Smith family after a short break in treatment. The family had been referred because of the middle child's hysterical epileptic episodes which had no organic foundation. After a few sessions with the whole family, these symptoms abated and did not return, but mother was immediately hospitalised for a psychotic breakdown. After her discharge, the therapists re-commenced sessions with the husband and wife and began intensive work on their marital problems. Amongst other difficulties it had been noted that a repeated escalation of tension occurred within the group, surrounding the husband's catatonic-like passivity. At first this was expressed by the middle child, but after treatment began, the combat between repression and explosion became centred within the marital pair and was expressed through the wife's bizarre explosive outbursts. In this extract, both the therapists and the marital pair are focusing on their minute-by-minute feelings of nervousness due to being observed through a one-way screen. If we as therapists had denied our own anxiety we would have been refusing to express or struggle with our own uncomfortable feelings, whilst expecting George and Joan to be able to do so. More importantly, we would have missed the opportunity of inching forward in our understanding of how each person coped with stress so differently. Sometimes the extract seems strained and halting; at other times, rambling and disjointed. But gradually, from examining the way in which the current anxiety is being dealt with, the group begins to move into important areas of work concerning Joan's easy ability to express caring for others and her inability to be cared for herself—a problem which both sustains and is sustained by the opposite dilemma experienced by her husband.

The group come into the interviewing room and take their seats as follows: Joan with her back to the observers, George opposite her, face on to the screen and the two therapists opposite each other.

| | |
|---|---|
| *Family Therapist (1):* | 'Would you prefer to be where you can half-see them [the observers] instead?' |
| *Joan:* | [Inaudible mutter and nervous laugh] |
| *Family Therapist (2):* | 'What did you say? [pause] You would rather not see them at all?' |
| *Joan:* | [Laughs] 'No!' |
| *F.T. (1):* | 'A bit like an ostrich! If he doesn't look maybe the danger won't be there!' |
| *F.T. (2):* | [to George] 'Do you mind being face on to the danger?' |
| *George:* | 'No, no.' |
| *Joan:* | 'Oh, they are not dangerous!' |
| *F.T. (1):* | 'What's a better word; that was my word.' |
| *Joan:* | 'I don't know—strangers, perhaps?' |
| *F.T. (1):* | 'Mm.' |
| *Joan:* | 'Yes?' |
| *F.T. (2):* | 'Well, they are strangers.' |
| *Joan:* | 'I'm making everybody feel terrible now!' |
| *F.T. (1):* | 'There is no reason why we shouldn't spread the feelings [of anxiety] round a bit.' [Pause] |
| *F.T. (2):* | 'If they are strangers to you two, if they are not dangerous, what do they make you feel inside now?' |
| *Joan:* | 'Just uncomfortable really. To be talking now while they are all there.' |
| *F.T. (2):* | 'Mm. hmm.' |
| *Joan:* | 'Do you know what I mean?' |
| *F.T. (2):* | 'Mm. Yes. Hmm. [Pause] It makes *me* feel *anxious*—that's the word I would use for *me*. But they make *you* feel *uncomfortable?*' |
| *Joan:* | 'Yes, just a bit.' |
| *F.T. (1):* | 'What Sue, in a way, is saying is that it's not just some uncomfortableness or whatever for you, it's for all of us—maybe for them over there as well, but certainly for us as a group . . .' |
| *George:* | 'Yes.' |

| | |
|---|---|
| *F.T. (1):* | ' . . . rather than just for you. It isn't simply that you are the "patient" who is the un-comfortable one.' |
| *George:* | 'It's like being on television.' |
| *F.T. (1):* | 'Aha?' |
| *George:* | 'In a way—and they are the audience.' |
| *F.T. (1):* | 'Have you ever been on television?' |
| *George:* | 'Only once.' |
| *Joan:* | 'That was his high spot, that was. I've got the photographs so that he can show them.' [She laughs] |
| *F.T. (1):* | 'Was that with you, or with somebody else?' |
| *Joan:* | 'Oh, no.' |
| *George:* | 'No, that was before we met. They gave us some "pep" pills, well, tranquillisers, before we went on.' |
| *F.T. (2):* | [Laughs] |
| *F.T. (1):* | 'Different from what we do!' |
| *F.T. (2):* | 'I guess it might be a good idea some of the time!' |
| *F.T. (1):* | [To co-therapist] 'For us, or for them, or for all of us?' |
| *F.T. (2):* | 'I can only talk for me!' [Pause] |
| *George:* | 'It's a job to break the ice, isn't it?' [Pause] |
| *F.T. (2):* | 'In a way we have laid some of our feelings of uncomfortableness on the table—I wonder how we can help each other, or ourselves, to deal with them? Perhaps we have already helped ourselves to deal with them, but [pause]—well—how do we look at this amongst the four of us?' |
| *Joan:* | 'Well, the last time I felt better as soon as we started talking.' |
| *F.T.(2):* | 'Mm. hmm. Yes.' [Pause for about a minute] |
| *Joan:* | 'We seem to have been following the same pattern lately, don't we? [to George].' [Pause] |
| *George:* | 'Joan's been saying that she would like to go back to work when she's fit again—she gets a bit bored at home all the time.' |
| *F.T. (2):* | 'Joan's brought this up several times, hasn't she?' |

| | |
|---|---|
| *George:* | 'Probably be a good thing.' |
| *F.T. (1):* | 'As far as we can work it out, is this an optimistic thing, with you looking forward to feeling near to being able to be who you usually are, and that includes being at work?' |
| *Joan:* | 'Mm. hmm. I want to go back into the solicitor's office again.' |
| *F.T. (1):* | 'Mm. hmm.' |
| *Joan:* | 'The work is so interesting there.' [Pause] 'Really and truly, I'd like to do nursing, but I have to wait for that . . . really . . . until they are just that little bit bigger, because the hours will be varied.' |
| *F.T.(1):* | 'Mm. hmm.' [Pause] |
| *F.T. (1):* | 'The bell that rings in my mind is that we are back on this "helping" and "being helped" theme which turned up once or twice last week, and again now.' |
| *George and Joan:* | 'Mm. hmm.' [Pause] |
| *Joan:* | 'I did go and see the Matron at the Hospital . . . [pause] . . . and she thought that I would be the kind of person that would like nursing, but she would advise me to leave it until the children are, you know, able . . . Millicent is seven now, so in another year or so, perhaps she will be big enough.' |
| *F.T. (1):* | 'We are very much in the future today, aren't we?' |
| *George:* | 'Yes . . . yes.' |
| *F.T. (2):* | 'Is this because the present was so difficult to look at . . . you know, I was thinking when you were saying "I am going to see if I can do some work that involves caring for others, and . . . " you were the person who first of all voiced here today the uncomfortableness in yourself, but found it difficult to go on then and say "Help me deal with the uncomfortableness". But on the other hand, you helped *us* deal with our uncomfortableness. You did some of the caring for us, by taking upon yourself the business of expressing it.' |

| | |
|---|---|
| F.T. (1): | 'Yes, and she made a sort of bridge between us and the observers, she was the one who turned round and. . . .' |
| George: | 'Yes . . . mm.' |
| F.T. (1): | 'Sue is saying you are good at being a nurse here to us. Is that because it's a way of trying to deal with your own feelings of wanting to be nursed . . . cared for yourself?' |

Defining a small piece of interaction with which to work is done by the family itself; all the therapist has to do is to 'freeze' the sequence long enough to extract the maximum therapeutic potential. The problem may be defined, by the description given by one family member, in passing, of some seemingly inconsequential exchange between family members—such as the row that took place over who was to drive the car to come to the session today. Or, it may be in the form of a non-verbal sequence which the therapist picks up from within the session itself. The purpose is always to help family members to examine these small interactive sequences and to try to work them through to a different conclusion. If a well-worn circular conflict can be broken, using an apparently trivial incident, family members can often move on to try out the same procedure with more obdurate transactional patterns in which they are caught. The following example is taken from a session with the Brown family consisting of Idris, aged 32, his wife, Gwyneth, aged 29, and their two children, Terry, aged 8 and Baby Darren, aged 6 months. The family was beset by a multiplicity of problems, some of them environmental and some interpersonal. The problem which was first presented to us was Gwyneth's inability to touch or to physically care for her son, Terry, who was severely mentally and physically handicapped. Her revulsion from her son was in strong contrast to her devotion to the baby and was so extreme that after a few days, or perhaps a week at home, he had to be hospitalised due to his state of physical neglect. Each time Terry was hospitalised, Idris and Gwyneth would have violent rows; Idris would stay out drinking every evening and Gwyneth would refuse to leave the house, blaming and punishing herself for her inability to care for Terry. Whilst Gwyneth was obviously greatly distressed by what she felt was her blameworthy neglect of Terry, it materialised that as a consequence of her guilty feelings, she would refuse to have intercourse with Idris, or to give or receive from him any physical caring. Thus the difficulties between Idris and Gwyneth escalated until Terry returned home and the cycle began again. It seemed that on an unconscious level, there were some secondary gains for Gwyneth at the point when she could start to punish herself for her neglect of Terry, as it turned out that her distaste of physical touch was more generalised than it first seemed, and in particular involved her physical relationship with her husband. Idris for his part was able to blame his wife for breaking up the family and 'causing' him to start drinking again, to stay away from home and to lose his job. Hence, when Terry was taken into hospital, Gwyneth had the 'excuse' to break off sexual relationships with her husband and he, to leave home and fly from the pressures of trying to provide a sufficient income for his dependants. Both Idris and Gwyneth therefore had something to gain from Gwyneth's phobia. In this session, the therapists are working with the general problem of intimacy experienced within the group and the way in which each family member becomes a barrier, standing in the way of intimacy developing between others. In this extract, the therapists are trying to re-define this general problem within the family in terms of the actual physical positions of family members in the session—and trying to get the family to experiment with reducing the physical gaps between them in the session as a stepping stone towards reducing them emotionally within their relationships.

*1st Therapist:* 'Do you both get the feeling that I get? Gwyneth said earlier today that "What I want from him, is him, himself" and you come in and say "What I want from her is herself, her to love me".'

*2nd Therapist:* 'You're saying the same exactly. You're saying the same things about each other exactly, but somehow they're on different levels. You can't come together on this.'

*1st Therapist:* [To co-therapist] 'What is it that goes wrong here?'

*2nd Therapist:* 'It's a block; it's like the space between them now.'

*Idris:* 'Well, I think I can take the blame there, it's a question of . . . '

*1st Therapist:* 'There's no question of blame.'

*Idris:* 'Let's try it this way then. When I come home from work next week, let's see if she can sort of break down the barrier, and come to terms.'

*1st Therapist:* 'Have we got to wait until next week? We can start from now.'

*Idris:* 'Well, let's start from now.'

*1st Therapist:* 'Yes, this very minute *now*. How could you get near each other now?'

*Idris:* 'Now? This minute?'

| | |
|---|---|
| *1st Therapist:* | 'Yes, now, this very minute.' |
| *Idris:* | 'Now? Don't know . . . [pause]. Just show affection, that's all I want.' |
| *1st Therapist:* | 'O.K. what would you like her to do to show affection?' |
| *Idris:* | 'Make a cup of tea. [Laughs] [Pause] I don't know. I don't want her slobbering all over me, and that's a fact, but, you know, as I says to David [the 2nd therapist] all I want her to do is talk to me with affection, instead of her demanding way.' |
| *2nd Therapist:* | 'Can I ask if there's anything *you* can do? We've talked about what Gwyneth can do for you, but what can you do for Gwyneth, now, in the same way?' |
| *Idris:* | 'I don't know.' |
| *1st Therapist:* | 'Well, let's turn it round the other way. We take the point that we're here and that makes a difference, but is there something that prevents you getting near to Idris? How can you get near to Idris and show him and get from him the sort of love that you each want? You've been saying to Idris: "You're never here, you never talk to me". Now he is here—so how can you show him the sort of love that he says he wants? What prevents you?' |
| *Gwyneth:* | [To Idris] 'Well, you're not here long enough to show it.' |
| *1st Therapist:* | 'But he's here now, this very minute.' |
| *Gwyneth:* | 'Now?' |
| *Idris:* | 'She's too shy. [Turning to Gwyneth] Give us a kiss then—and let's make up.' |
| | [Idris moves hesitantly towards Gwyneth on the settee, but Gwyneth draws away, prompting Idris to quickly withdraw too] |
| *Idris:* | [Cynically] 'Well, give us a kiss for two bob, then.' |
| *Gwyneth:* | [Sadly] 'We're too old.' |
| | [At this point, Terry interrupts with a loud long drawn out, animal-like noise. Idris mimics the noise and then says to Terry 'Do you love Mamma? No. Shove her out of your mind, Son. Shove her out of your mind'. At the point at which Idris and Gwyneth attempt to get a bit closer physically and emotionally in the session, Terry interrupts and Idris uses the interruption defensively as a direct distancing reaction to the tentative movement he had made towards his wife.] |

58

## Behavioural approaches[2]

In a general sense, many of the family therapists' treatment
interventions could be described as reinforcement of desired
behaviour, but techniques utilised by some therapists are derived
more consciously from those of behaviour modification. Viewed
from the standpoint of learning theory, family members' responses
to the dysfunctional behaviour of, for example, the identified
patient, has the effect of reinforcing his deviance, maintaining and
even increasing it. Because this family member's behaviour has
often come to hold such an hypnotic effect for everyone in the group,
the behaviour of the rest of the family by way of attention and punishment has a correspondingly powerful impact on the subject. No one
seems to be able to remember anything else happening during the
week at home except Johnnie's temper tantrums and the effect these
have upon everyone else. Thus the message received by Johnnie is
that so long as he continues having his temper tantrums, everyone
will be interested in him (even though this interest is expressed by
anger, punishment, tears, etc.) and he will remain the centre of the
family's attention. Once this pattern of response has been 'learned',
only infrequent doses of reinforcement are needed to maintain the
behaviour. Because of the reciprocal nature of family processes,
mutual reinforcement takes place between family members. Hence,
mother may be able to abate Johnnie's tantrum by giving him a bag
of sweets—the ensuing peace and quiet reinforcing her inappropriate
compliance with his demands. The family therapist who uses
techniques derived from learning theory seeks to teach family
members to break through this cycle of mutual reinforcement and
instead, to reinforce other, more desirable behavioural expressions
which family members find pleasing. The therapist assumes the role
of educator and instructs family members directively as to how to
change their ways of behaving towards each other. His task as a
family therapist is to intervene and change the family's *reciprocal
reinforcing patterns,* not merely to use one family member as a
therapist to change the behaviour of the identified patient. In
addition, the therapist acts as a role model to family members in the
way in which he reinforces, by his approval, their attempts to comply
with the agreed behaviour changes. As with task-centred work (to be
discussed in greater detail in the next chapter) family therapists who
use learning theory often find it helpful to use role-playing and
simulation exercises within the session to enable family members to
experiment with the new behaviour patterns.
    The following provides a case example of the use of a behavioural
approach in family therapy. The family consisted of husband (Jack)
aged 42, wife (Geraldine) aged 27, Patty, aged 10, Michael, aged 5

and Baby Louise. Patty was Jack's child by his first wife, whilst Michael and Louise were the children of the current marriage. The family was referred because of Geraldine's suspected ill-treatment of Patty, who regularly arrived at school with a black eye, or bruised legs. During the course of the early meetings with this family it materialised that Geraldine hated and resented Patty because she was the child of her husband's first wife. She felt insecure in her position as Jack's second wife and could not tolerate the continual reminder which Patty provided. She complained bitterly of being merely a housekeeper, and an unpaid one at that. It materialised, however, that Jack started out in business on his own soon after they married, and spent most of his working life running the business. For relaxation he would enjoy television and then retire to bed to sleep soundly till morning. The only time he gave his wife or the children his undivided attention was when she began shouting at Patty. He would then stop everything he was doing and rush toward her to prevent her from hitting the child. He would then go to comfort Patty, who had discovered that by irritating her stepmother, she would ultimately gain her father's attention. Geraldine's hatred and rejection of Patty thus received continual re-inforcement—as this was the only time that either she or Patty were attended to or comforted by Jack. The therapist suggested that each member of this triangle change their behaviour in relation to the others in the following ways. Jack would try to take the initiative in appreciating Geraldine's daily domestic activities, when he returned from work. He would comment positively on the way she had cared for the flat and on the meal she had prepared. Geraldine would respond favourably to her husband's advances, reinforcing by her approval the efforts that he was making. In particular, she would endeavour to maintain this response consistently, as one of Jack's complaints about Geraldine was the way in which she would 'blow hot and cold' towards him unpredictably. Patty would make a point of taking her torn or damaged clothes to Geraldine as soon as the accident had occurred—as one of the main irritants for Geraldine was the way in which Patty hid the damage until Geraldine discovered it too late to salvage. Jack would spend at least quarter of an hour each evening with Patty, talking over what she had done at school and sharing in her interests with her. He would also refrain from getting involved with the rows that took place between Geraldine and Patty, so that this attention-seeking behaviour by both females would not be reinforced. In this way all three members of the triangle could be assured of the approval of the others without having to extract it forceably by dysfunctional behaviour. The family had to struggle with achieving these interlocking behaviour changes over a period of months, but gradually the focus of treatment shifted away from the dysfunctional relationship between Geraldine and Patty and work continued with the marital pair.

## Mechanical aids

The use of mechanical aids deserves the attention of family therapists since, quite apart from their usefulness in learning and teaching, they can be employed as powerful tools by the therapist in the course of treatment. It may be objected that such equipment is costly and that one can hardly expect it to be placed high on an agency's list of priorities, when many social workers have to work without the help of even a suitable interviewing room. However, an increasing number of probation and social service departments as well as hospital social work units (especially in the larger teaching hospitals) do have access to audio tape-recorders, video taping equipment and/or to a one-way viewing screen. For this reason, it seems worth giving some attention to the varying uses of audio-visual aids in the treatment of the family group.

One of the therapist's tasks in both individual and family treatment is to enable the client to employ his 'observing ego' more fully and more functionally. Family members are assisted to become observers as well as participants in relation to their own interactions. One way of helping family members to 'step outside' the emotional impact of an interchange is to ask them to 'step outside' literally, by going behind a one-way viewing screen (Minuchin *et al.,* 1967). Where co-therapists are working together, one therapist may accompany the family member and discuss with him his perceptions as an observer, whilst the other therapist continues working with the rest of the family. This can be a particularly useful technique to employ early in treatment with the identified patient. It takes him out of the 'hot seat' and makes it possible for one of the therapists to form a strong alliance with him. If the identified patient is a child, he may feel much freer in talking about his painful feelings while watching his parents and siblings interact without him. This experience may also give him the feeling for the first time that, despite what his family are continually telling him, he is not the source of all their unhappiness. If, for example, the identified patient is having difficulties in separating from his family, he may begin to realise, while experiencing the partial separation afforded by the screen, that his family will not fall apart if he leaves them and, even though his parents have rows, he does not have to remain at home to prevent them from destroying each other. Each movement in and out of the room changes the composition of the group and the dynamics of interaction. The screen can be used by the therapist as a semi-permeable membrane, to break up coalitions and to re-align pairings. It may, for example, be useful at a particular stage in treatment to invite an especially destructive family member to go behind the screen. This will serve the dual purpose of enabling the rest of the family to interact with each other and with the remaining therapist more freely, whilst, at the same time, enabling the second therapist to get alongside the destructive member, perhaps freeing him to exercise other aspects of his personality. Such manoeuvres can of course be used defensively by the therapist. The aim must always be to assist family members to struggle with the hard task of conflict resolution face to face with each other; the therapist and his tools are only means to achieving that end. As with every other therapeutic technique, timing is the touchstone of its utility.

When working with a highly enmeshed family, the therapist may find it helpful to separate the fused relationships and enable significant pairings such as husband and wife, father and daughter, father and son, etc., to have the opportunity of communicating with each other without using the defensive manoeuvre of triangling in a third person, to syphon off emotional pressure from the dyad. Each of the other family members can be taught, from the other side of the screen, to become observers to the interaction of other sub-groupings, thus allowing them the opportunity of achieving both greater intimacy and greater differentiation. Used in this way, the one-way screen provides opportunities different from those of the separate interview offered to sub-groupings within the system. The screen allows sufficient separation to enable family members to experiment with some differentiation, but it maintains the essential wholeness of the treatment situation, with participants and observers remaining in dynamic interaction with each other.

Audio and video recordings offer therapist and family members different opportunities, for both have the unique advantage of allowing instant replay of any part of the therapy session.[3] It may be that the therapist has noted a circular communication pattern occurring frequently between two family members. Instead of commenting on the pattern, he may feel it to be less threatening and more impactful, simply to play back the few moments of tape-recording which contain the sequence. Family members usually feel the impact of actually hearing (or seeing) themselves more powerfully than they do the therapist's subjective description of how he experiences their interaction. In fact, it is often more useful to play back the extract without comment, leaving family members to draw their own conclusions. In this way, responsibility for seeking out and changing dysfunctional behaviour patterns is placed firmly back upon the family + therapist group as a whole, rather than seeming to reside in the therapist alone.

It is sometimes useful to arrange a series of sessions whereby the therapist alternates a videotaped session with one which is devoted to the playback of the previous interview in its entirety. This enables the family to gain the maximum feedback which the videotape can provide. It is a useful way of working with families that have a fragile corporate identity—where perhaps one or more family members has been absent for long periods of time in hospital, prison or children's home. The repeated visual impact of the video picture helps to build up the family's sense of its own boundary and its identity as a group. More often, the therapist will use small pieces of tape to play back to the family. It has been found that where the 'image impact' of seeing the picture is marked, either positively or negatively, treatment outcome is more hopeful than when family members react with indifference. Thus, therapists have experimented with different ways of selecting the piece of tape to be shown in order to maximise its impact. Sometimes 'focused re-play' is used, whereby the extract is carefully selected by the therapist to fit the family's particular phase of treatment; at other times, the extract has been selected randomly either by the therapist or by a family member. Both methods have different advantages: the first allows the therapist to select extracts which will contribute most helpfully to the overall treatment process, from his unique vantage point as therapist; the second enables all family members to take an active part in selecting a sequence, which may have particular meaning for them (Berger, 1970).

Since so much of a family's communication is non-verbal, it is obviously more useful to use a video tape-recording, so that family members and therapist can watch as well as hear. Fundamental discrepancies between verbal content and non-verbal metacommunication will often become quickly apparent to the family. However, few of us at present are able to make use of video recordings as more than an occasional tool—whereas a small audio tape-recorder is often more readily available, and will provide an enormous amount of unique data for the therapist to use with the family. A particular advantage of audio-taping is that family members can take away the tape of an important session and re-play it over to themselves at home. In this way, the tape can act as a 'reinforcer' for the family during the period between sessions.

If the family is to feel confident and re-assured as to the potential usefulness of these aids, the therapist must first feel confident himself. This means that he must be prepared to be confronted, along with the family, with his own self-image; but in the case of the therapist, he must also be prepared to be confronted by the lacunae and inadequacies in his own therapeutic technique. For most of us, this is not easy. And yet, both audio and video recordings, and the one-way viewing screen can be invaluable resources for the therapist to employ in his own struggle for increased self-awareness. Particularly when he feels that he has exhausted his efforts and reached stalemate, he will find it invaluable to invite a colleague to observe a session from behind the screen. If the therapist is struggling to disentangle himself from some blocking counter-transference resonance, it may be more appropriate for the consultant/observer to offer the therapist his thoughts after the family has left. On other occasions, it may be helpful for the whole family + therapist group to meet with the observer for the last few minutes of the session and for his 'feedback' to be offered to the whole group. Again, the therapist may find it helpful from time to time to arrange with the family for the observer to come into the interviewing room whenever he feels that the process is becoming side-tracked. This procedure may help therapist and family to experience a greater degree of unity in their mutual commitment to the treatment goals. The outsider can facilitate communication between them and in this way assist them as a total group.

## The course of treatment

In family therapy, as in other types of psycho-social treatment, 'there is no magic and there are no magicians' (Pittman, 1973). Moreover, there is no one right way to do family therapy. This being the case, the setbacks, resistances and other vicissitudes which confront the therapist during the normal course of treatment are infinitely various and can be handled in many different ways. The length of treatment which the therapist proposes undertaking will affect the timing and manifestation of some of the familiar landmarks which occur during the treatment process. And a decision as to the length of treatment will depend upon what the therapist hopes and expects to achieve. First, if he is working mainly with families in a *state of acute crisis,* with one or more members requiring immediate hospitalisation, his overall objective may simply be to return the family to its pre-crisis *'status quo',* without resorting to hospitalisation, and the length of treatment may be reduced to the few weeks during which the family actually remains in crisis. Crisis, whether occurring in an individual or a family group, can be defined as an acute state of disequilibrium, brought about by a reaction to internal or external stress factors. Langsley, Kaplan and Pittman *et al.* (1967) have delineated seven phases which occur in the course of this type of family crisis therapy: the initial response to emergency; re-definition of the crisis in terms of the family system; focusing the dimensions of the current situation; relief of anxiety and abatement of symptomatology; encouragement of problem-solving activities, including task assignments; negotiation around resistances to change; and termination. Because of the transitory nature of a crisis situation, the therapist emphasises a strictly problem-oriented approach and works towards limited, clearly defined goals. (Such an approach has been advocated for use by the intake teams in Social Service Departments, since it is likely to involve the worker in only rapid, short-term work, as well as potentially averting the necessity for removing one or more family members into hospital, children's home, or temporary accommodation (Loewenstein, 1974)). Other workers have found that even one or two family therapy sessions offered at a crisis point can be far-reaching in their therapeutic effects (Skynner, 1969a).

Second, some family therapists specialise in offering *brief intervention,* which may or may not be crisis linked. Brief intervention is usually conducted over a period of up to six months and then terminated. The number of sessions is usually fixed, regardless of the type or severity of the presenting symptom. For example, at the Brief Therapy Centre, Mental Research Institute, California, workers offer a maximum number of ten sessions, usually on a weekly basis (Weakland *et al.,* 1974). Like those engaged in family crisis therapy, this group delineates several specific phases of treatment and uses the constraints imposed by the limited time-scale as a positive promoter of change. Alternatively, brief intervention may be offered as part of a pattern of treatment periods interspersed by carefully timed periods of recession. During the recession the family integrates the work of the previous treatment period, before engaging in another series of sessions. The latter approach combines the advantages of brief intervention with those of a carefully planned follow-up procedure, and has been likened to the way in which a General Practitioner tries to maintain his patients at a general level of physical health within the community (Minuchin, 1974a). This approach helps the family to concentrate on working with manageable segments of their interpersonal problems and gives them space to integrate the work they have accomplished during the recession period without the danger of becoming dependent on the therapist's presence. At the follow-up interview, the therapist can determine with the family whether or not another series of sessions is required and if so, how the specific treatment goals for these should be defined. For example: during the first series of sessions the work may concentrate on getting some abatement in the presenting symptomatology of the child if he is the identified patient—especially when the symptom is grossly incapacitating or endangers the life of the child. If this has been successfully accomplished, the second series of sessions may be directed towards a different sub-system, such as the marital pair and will focus upon the difficulties within the marriage. Even though an intensive period of work may be required at the beginning, this is, nevertheless, an economical method of work and makes use of the period of recession, when the therapist is not meeting with the family, as an integral part of the treatment process. When using brief intervention, therapists normally arrange sessions at frequent intervals, perhaps two or three times a week, especially at the outset of treatment. This enables therapist and family to maximise the potential offered by the acute situation. Thus, brief intervention commends itself to many therapists, not as a 'second best' arrangement but as the treatment of choice, simply because, in family therapy, even quite complex interpersonal problems can often be worked through much more quickly than in individual work.

Third, the family therapist may choose to work for much longer periods with some of his families and will expect to achieve a more fundamental re-organisation within the family system. When treatment continues for a year or more, the phases that normally occur during the treatment process are more clearly worked out. After the difficulties which usually surround engagement, when the family is manifesting primary resistance towards viewing their difficulties as a family concern, the newly formed group of family + family therapist often enter a 'honeymoon' period. Overt symptomatology improves, or sometimes abates altogether and both the therapist and the family seem pleased with each other's efforts. The group then invariably encounters secondary resistances which may be manifested by a deepening dependence upon the therapist, who finds himself increasingly pushed to take the initiative and produce motivation for continued work and change. Family and therapist become bored with each other. More alarmingly, a series of critical incidents may begin to occur during which family members throw up their hands in despair and blame the therapist and/or themselves for the fact that 'nothing has changed really'. The critical incident which takes place may seem quite bizarre and uncharacteristic, such as a suicidal gesture or the beginnings of divorce proceedings or rapid decompensation on the part of a marginally involved family member, all of which can be very alarming for the therapist as well as for the family. During this phase, the identified patient, who was instrumental in bringing the family into treatment in the first place, may begin to back-pedal and apparently lead the family in its flight from the therapist. This is not surprising when we remember the secondary gains which the identified patient usually derives from his position, however uncomfortable this position may seem to be to an outsider. For example: a child who was refusing to attend school because of his half-conscious fears that, if he left his mother's side, she would walk out on the family, may have become sufficiently reassured during the first few sessions, to attend school regularly. However, at the point when his parents begin successfully to tackle the increasing gap within their marital relationship, the child may begin to feel excluded from his mother's side, following the greater degree of closeness being experienced within the marital relationship. The child may at this point react by reverting to his previous symptomatology and refusing to attend school or by manifesting his unhappiness via other attention-seeking behaviour. Alternatively, another child in the family, who had previously been a-symptomatic, may react unfavourably to the changes in his parents' relationship and may become the new identified patient. Hence symptom exchange during this phase in treatment is not unusual. The occurrence of a critical incident is not, however, necessarily a negative feature of the treatment process. It may presage a new release of energy within the family and its successful handling can be converted by the therapist into a means of accelerating change. It may represent 'a desperate reaching out towards the therapist, but often in a secret, not fully conscious manner' (Boszormenyi-Nagy, 1970).

The middle phases of treatment are usually characterised by a steady ebb and flow in the pace of movement and growth. Resistance, both conscious and unconscious, continues to be a normal reaction to the pain and anxiety engendered by change. It is inevitably more complex than the resistance which occurs in the treatment of individuals and can take a variety of forms.[4] Sometimes a key member of the treatment group will refuse to come to sessions, or the whole family will state its intention to terminate treatment prematurely. It is usually fruitless for the therapist to engage in any head-on collision with family members who are threatening to do this. Instead he should try to manoeuvre for compromise, perhaps suggesting that sessions be halted for a while. If the therapist opens up this option, the family will often reciprocate by agreeing to an early follow-up date. Resistance can be expressed by family members refusing to undertake any of the changes in their interactional patterns which could alleviate their problems. They come regularly and obediently to the sessions, but hold on doggedly to their distress. When confronted with this situation, it may be useful for the *therapist* to use the threat to terminate treatment prematurely, unless the family is prepared to offer some response. This technique is sometimes remarkably effective—maybe because of the oppositional relationship which already exists between family and therapist, and which encourages family members to start changing *despite* the therapist (Zuk, 1971).

If the therapist is employing the type of intermittent work described earlier, whereby treatment is interspersed by periods of recession, the concept of termination is inappropriate. Working in this way, the family therapist's services can be thought of as an ongoing resource, to be used in times of crisis or special need. In this context there is no termination in the usual sense, for the family carries with it, more or less continuously, the image of the family therapist, even when he is physically absent for long periods of time.

However, in most types of work, the terminal phases of family therapy are marked by a progressive disengagement on the part of the therapist and the removal of the boundary which has held the family + therapist group together during treatment. If treatment has been extensive, the termination of the relationship between family and therapist needs careful preparation and may include periods of 'trial separation' during which intervals between sessions are progressively lengthened. Family groups will react differently to termination, some by becoming markedly more dependent, requesting more sessions and 'discovering' more problems. Others will perceive termination as a rejection on the part of the therapist and will terminate angrily and prematurely as an attempt at avoiding the pain of separation. The therapist often needs help from his colleagues in dealing with his own ambivalent feelings. He may feel relieved that work with a demanding family is ending, and yet feel guilty about his relief. He may, on the other hand, find himself deferring the decision to terminate when he finds a family enjoyable to work with and unconsciously he increases their dependency on him. Families will often terminate after a specific piece of emotional work has been completed even though the therapist may feel doubtful that change will be sustained without a more prolonged period of treatment. It is worth remembering, however, that the family therapist's mandate is to help to create the minimum amount of re-organisation needed to support enduring improvement. The roots of the family's emotional well-being need to be firmly established; but the therapist need only dig as deeply as is required to secure them.

## Notes

1 Goldstein (1973). In chapter 3, the author lists several studies which have assessed the importance of workers' style as a variable in practice.
2 Accounts of behavioural approaches used within a family psychotherapeutic approach are given by Liberman (1972) and Azrin *et al.* (1973).
3 Different ways of using audio-visual aids are discussed by Alger and Hogan (1970); Stoller (1970); and Alger (1973).
4 The many different forms which resistance can take in family therapy are discussed in Soloman (1969).

# Chapter six

# Task-centred family therapy

'I'm afraid you've not had much practice in riding' Alice
ventured to say, as she helped him up from his fifth tumble.
The Knight looked very much surprised, and a little offended at
the remark. 'What makes you say that?' he asked, as he
scrambled back into the saddle, keeping hold of Alice's hair
with one hand, to save himself from falling over on the other
side. 'Because people don't fall off quite so often, when they've
had much practice.'

Lewis Carroll, *Through the Looking Glass*

Task-centred family therapy involves a highly structured approach
towards changing the dysfunctional family system. The dysfunctional
family can be compared to a group of actors who have got stuck. The
first scenes have been over-rehearsed—yet their play cannot be
completed. The family therapist enters this situation in a dual role;
he becomes a new actor in the play and he becomes, too, the stage
director of the total experience. In this second capacity, he must be
prepared to direct the production in an active, involving way, until
fusion has occurred between the actor's own self and that of the
character he is attempting to portray (Kantor and Hoffman, 1966).

Like all analogies, this one must break down eventually—but it
indicates some important aspects of the task-centred approach.
First, the family therapy session is a microcosmic expression of the
family's continuous drama, enacted during the other twenty-three
hours of the day, during which the therapist is not with them. It is
important, however, to distinguish between the functions of these two
juxtaposed groups—the family group on the one hand and the family
+ therapist group on the other. The family group must remain
responsible for its ongoing life but the therapist must take hold of
responsibility for the newly formed group of family + therapist—

like the director of a play. Carl Whitaker summarises the situation when he says that the therapist is responsible for the *therapy* and the family for *itself*. To put it another way—the family takes care of the 'what' and the therapist takes care of the 'how'. Second, the family therapy session is about re-enactment and experimentation—the re-enactment by the family of their dysfunctional communication patterns, followed by the family's attempts to experiment with new, adaptive patterns of response. The family therapist enables the session to be used for both these functions and the task-centred approach offers some powerful tools for helping him in this endeavour. This approach emphasises the fact that family therapy is primarily experiential and that the therapist is trying to establish the treatment session as a laboratory for the family to experiment with desired change. Third, those who advocate task-centred work emphasise the fact that family therapy is a problem-oriented rather than a method-oriented approach, and whilst the engagement period of the work may involve the family in some sort of re-definition of their original problem, it is nevertheless the therapist's job to help family members to engage successfully in the problem-solving activities which, prior to treatment, they have been unable to negotiate.

**Therapeutic tasks**

I would define a therapeutic task as used in this approach as follows:

The physical enactment of an emotional reality—either as a means of heightening the family's awareness of its existing dysfunctional relationships or as a means of restructuring those relationships to achieve the established treatment goals.

As a therapeutic tool, a task must first have a clearly defined *purpose* within the ongoing therapeutic process and must be timed as sensitively as a verbal interpretation used in traditional psycho-therapeutic methods. Second, it must be *practised* or tried out, either actually or symbolically within the therapy session itself and modified if necessary in order best to achieve the treatment goal. Third, it must be capable of being *performed* within the family's ongoing life outside the session—in other words, the experimenta-tion within the session must be transferred. These three 'P's— purpose, practice and performance, should be regarded as the hallmarks of a well constructed therapeutic task. Here it is important to note that the term *therapeutic* task is used to distinguish these tasks from an educative learning activity *per se*. A therapeutic task often has no intrinsic value in itself; its meaning lies in the symbolic restructuring of relationships which is attendant upon its performance. Moreover 'success' or 'failure' in the execution of tasks is not of primary significance to the therapist—since a well-constructed task involves different levels of the family's functioning—and the family will usually manage to succeed on one level, whilst failing on others. Again, the therapist is interested in the *how* of the matter. How has the family set about the task? Are different alliances and communication patterns beginning to appear within the family? Or are new levels of resistance making themselves felt? A comment by Montalvo (1973, p. 356) summarises the point:

> Tasks become not merely a way of defining events that must take place for change to occur, but ways of re-aligning relationships in a field of which [the therapist] is a part so as to facilitate change. He is thus restrained from assuming that his tasks address themselves to repairing problems of social incompetence, of ignorance or cognition.

Therapeutic tasks fall into two main types—those which are worked out *within* the therapy session and those which are constructed for the family to work on *between* sessions. The first type of internal task includes diagnostic procedures employed to recreate dysfunctional interaction or symptomatic behaviour within the session, and treatment interventions encouraging the family to try out something new. The second type of task, worked on externally by the family, can be thought of as a sort of homework assignment, suggested sometimes by the therapist, and sometimes (especially later on in treatment) by a family member.

## Case illustration

I will illustrate the use of these two types of tasks by referring to work undertaken with the Jones family over a period of three months. The family consisted of husband and wife in their late and middle 40s respectively; Lynne, 22 years, who had left home to teach physical education; Sarah, 21 years, the identified patient, who had become anorectic; Andrew, 18 years, who had tried living with his girlfriend briefly but was now back home without a job; and Colin, aged 10 years.

In Bowen's terms (1971), the Jones family can be described as having an undifferentiated ego mass, typical of a highly enmeshed family. There were weak, almost non-existent boundaries around the marital pair; confusion in the generational boundaries and little differentiation between them; mixed up sexual identification with unresolved oedipal conflicts; little or no dyadic transactions, and if these did occur, they concerned a third person who, instead of creating a triadic transaction, should more appropriately have been

71

engaged in the original dyad; communication patterns and activities tended to be triadic or group, with a third or more persons always getting involved in issues rightly belonging to a dyad. There was continual conflict in the family—but always of a parent-child nature, which served to hide the many unacknowledged husband/wife conflicts which existed. The family operated via a flight/fight defence amongst others, the male members in flight and the females in fight. Parents were allowed to 'blow their top' at children but not with each other, and the children were unable to argue with their parents. There was, therefore, a culture of conflict avoidance in the family into which Sarah's symptom of anorexia fitted. By becoming anorectic, she was able to be oppositional, but in a covert way. Her anorexia also served the purpose of absorbing the family's attention and concern, and enabling a buffer to be placed between the parents and their dysfunctional, potentially conflicting relationship. The secondary gains held by the symptom for the family were thus three-fold:

a   It gave Sarah a powerful means of confrontation, and changed her position within the family from that of extreme impotence to an unaccustomed powerfulness. It also enabled her to avoid having to confront the outside world, which was, she phantasised, full of powerful adults, like her parents. Her refusal to ingest the outside world through food, safeguarded her from having to reality test her phantasies concerning it.

b   It deflected energy and attention from the unresolved marital conflicts.

c   By scapegoating Sarah, Andrew could attain a reasonable degree of autonomy while his parents' attention was entirely taken up with Sarah. Thus, his 'health' depended upon Sarah's 'sickness'.

During the second session, the therapists arranged to offer the family a meal, consisting of a choice of snacks and hot drinks, thus enabling the family to recreate the symptomatic behaviour within the session. Since family therapy is about doing, rather than talking about doing, it made more sense for the therapists working with this family, to watch and take part with them in a meal, than simply to talk about eating.[1] More precisely, the therapists' own reactions to the emotional pressures within the system could be used as diagnostic clues to further their understanding of the dynamics involved. For example, during this meal, Sarah refused articles of food four times; she became noticeably stronger in relation to others in the group, being prepared to contribute verbally, she seemed less depressed compared with the earlier part of the session, but she also became more isolated within the group from the point when her eating difficulties became clearly demonstrated. While consciously wishing to align myself with Sarah and to refuse food, I was ultimately constrained to eat, by the powerful norm to conform which resided in this group. This norm became powerful on the parent-child axis, and since I experienced these parents transferentially as parents to me—I very soon succumbed. In this way, the therapists had an immediate experience of the way in which individuals needed to take extreme positions, such as anorexia, to break free of the undifferentiated family ego. Any less covert non-conformity carried high sanctions. In *our* handling of this task, we were employing the principle outlined by Minuchin (1974a) of using part of the family's defensive system to propel it towards change. In asking family members to eat, we asked them to re-enact in the session an occasion which held tension and difficulty for everyone, not only for Sarah, but we handled it differently from the family's usual obsession with each other's eating habits. During this meal, eating was not mentioned, and in particular Sarah's refusal to eat was ignored. The parents' attempts to draw our attention to Sarah were diverted and at this point in the treatment process, we adopted the position of confirming and reinforcing Sarah's choice to use food refusal as a primitive means of placing some boundary around herself as a separate, adult individual against her parents' intrusiveness. Our task as therapists is to render the presenting problem unnecessary, not to remove it prematurely, which can, and frequently does, lead to symptom exchange. Before it was safe for Sarah to eat, some major restructuring within the family's system of relationships had to be undertaken.

Did this meal fulfil the three requirements of a therapeutic task? Its two-fold *purpose* was to recreate the anorectic symptom within the session, and more fundamentally to engage with the family initially on its own terms around the symptom but to receive and use the symptom in such a way that the family could begin to use it as a springboard for growth instead of a defensive retreat. During the meal we modelled for the family members a different way of dealing with their anxiety, by refusing to discuss eating and instead, engaging in some exploration of the underlying conflicts concerning privacy and intrusion which lie behind the anorectic symptoms. We thus enabled the family members to *practise* in a tentative way what we later gave them as a task to be *performed* during their ongoing life together—an avoidance of all discussion and criticism of each other's eating habits.[2]

Towards the end of this session, we re-arranged the seating so that Sarah and Andrew sat together, and thus made the first move towards constructing an external task, which we suggested to the family during the later part of this session—some outside activity for Sarah and Andrew undertaken separately from the rest of the family group. In asking Sarah and Andrew to sit together during the remainder of the session, the therapists asked the family to *practise* re-defining its sub-groupings and to experience in a limited way some of the tensions and stress that this re-definition may cause them if the task is, in fact, performed during the following week. This gave the therapists the opportunity to notice, for example, Sarah's anxious look when her mother was asked to move from beside her to make way for Andrew, and to notice too, Andrew's hesitancy in responding to the suggestion to move close to his sister. In other words, the secondary gains which prompt family members to collude in the identified patient's predicament reveal themselves. In this way, some working through of potentially critical areas can be attempted during the session to strengthen the family against its own resistance towards *performing* the external task.

The rest of this session was thus taken up by the family discussing how to go about this task, and what feelings might be aroused by it in all family members.

Our *purpose* behind suggesting this external task, was two-fold:

First, it was a beginning attempt at firming up the generational boundaries and creating a clearer differentiation between the parents on the one hand, and the children on the other.

Second, it sought to distinguish and alter the sexual alliances which are confused along both a same sex and an oedipal dimension.

There existed, for example, a primary entrenched symbiosis between mother and Sarah, and a secondary, less intense symbiosis between father and Andrew. In constructing this task, the therapists were seeking to *use* the family's defence of symbiosis to propel the system towards change. We therefore prescribed change *within* the scope of the family's defensive myth of symbiotic pairings, and thus tried to prevent our change intervention from being perceived as too challenging and dangerous to the family system. Thus, the task suggests a pairing, but one which has to operate on one side of, instead of across, the generational boundary; and it further suggests that this pairing be of a heterosexual nature. Here we need to remember that a therapeutic task often has no intrinsic value in itself. In this case, there *would* be some secondary pay-off from Sarah achieving an outing apart from her parents (and the family no doubt saw this as the sole purpose) but the purpose of the task from the therapists' point of view, resided chiefly in the symbolic restructuring of alliances for which it provided a forerunner. Our goal was clearly not to create a permanent alliance for its own sake between Sarah and Andrew, who both need to move out of the family into their separate lives. But before they could begin to do this, there needed to be some re-integration between the split-off sick and healthy areas, which had been manifested in Sarah and Andrew separately. More important still, some re-integration brought about between Sarah and Andrew paves the way for the difficulties within the marital relationship to be exposed and worked on, and for therapeutic strategies to be devised for enabling David and Rita to become husband and wife again, instead of simply an over-functioning parental pair.

In the following extract, the family report failure of this task, on one level, but they use the session to try again.

| | |
|---|---|
| *Sarah:* | 'We haven't been on our outing . . . yet.' |
| *Andrew:* | 'Confessions! [pause] But we have decided what to do, haven't we?' |
| *Sarah:* | 'Well . . . yes, we have decided to go to the cinema, but the one film that is not just for children, because it is the holidays, is a film that Andrew has already seen.' |
| *Andrew:* | 'But I will see it again—I would love to see it again.' |
| *David:* | 'You mean, the film at the Odeon?' |
| *Sarah:* | 'But it is better to see something new. I'm not having you sitting there saying "It's boring, I've seen all this before!"' [General laughter] |
| *Andrew:* | 'I won't say anything—I would really like to see it again. I said I wanted to see it again, didn't I? [speaking to mother]' [Pause] |
| *Rita:* | 'Yes, oh yes. I'm sorry I didn't realise you were speaking to me. I was looking at Sarah.' |
| *First Therapist:* | [To Andrew] 'Do you need her as an ally?' |
| *Andrew:* | 'Well, Sarah probably just thinks I am *saying* that I would like to see the film again, but I'm not, I would really like to see it again. Is it on tonight?' |
| *David:* | [Laughs] 'I am fascinated listening to you keep saying "I'd like to see it again; I'd like to see it again." Where is the money coming from to go, I wonder?' |
| *Rita:* | 'Well, I am holding his money at the moment.' |
| *David:* | 'In that case you owe me £1.30 already.' |
| *First Therapist:* | 'Sarah led us firmly into work and then Andrew began to look at the task and then he sidled away.' |

| | |
|---|---|
| *Andrew:* | [To Mother] 'You owe me £1!' |
| *First Therapist:* | [To Andrew] 'You are sidling away.' |
| *Andrew:* | 'I just thought I'd point that out.' |
| *First Therapist:* | 'Well, you have either got to convince Sarah, haven't you, that it is an enjoyable thing for you to go and see this film, and that you are not going to tell her the plot, um, one minute in advance as it unravels, or you have got to try to work out something else to do together.' |
| *Andrew:* | 'Well, I don't mind going to see it.' |
| *David:* | [To Sarah] 'Have you read the book?' |
| *Sarah:* | 'No, I don't know anything about it.' |
| *Andrew:* | 'I think you would enjoy it and find it very funny actually.' |
| *David:* | [To Andrew] 'Have you still got the book?' |
| *Andrew:* | 'Yes, somewhere.' |
| *First Therapist:* | [To David] 'What is the point you are making?' |
| *David:* | 'Well, in case Sarah would be tempted to read the book before going. But you wouldn't, would you? [to Sarah] She is very strong willed over some things [addressed to First Therapist].' |
| *First Therapist:* | 'Why should she not look at the book if she wants to?' |
| *David:* | 'I don't know. Nothing to stop her, I suppose, except that I think it takes the, er, the er, the interest away from the film, if she has already read the book.' |
| *First Therapist:* | 'Mm. Well, it would for you. But you are assuming that it would also take away from the enjoyment for Sarah. You are back to "knowing" how she feels.' |
| *David:* | [Angrily] 'I was just leading Sarah into a discussion.' |
| *First Therapist:* | 'But that is not the issue, is it, between these two [pointing to Andrew and Sarah].' |
| *Sarah:* | 'I would rather see the film without looking at the book. I am not a great reader anyway. I just find people's expressions . . . I just find watching things much more interesting than reading.' |
| *First Therapist:* | 'Mm. Mm. Yes.' |
| *Second Therapist:* | 'But you would also like Andrew to come fresh to the film as well?' |
| *Sarah:* | 'Yes, I think so.' |
| *First Therapist:* | 'Could you tell him why?' |
| *Sarah:* | 'Well, it would probably be a nicer outing for |

|                    |                                                                                                                                                                                                                                                                                                                                                                                                                                                                                                                                                                                                                                                                                                                |
| ------------------ | ---------------------------------------------------------------------------------------------------------------------------------------------------------------------------------------------------------------------------------------------------------------------------------------------------------------------------------------------------------------------------------------------------------------------------------------------------------------------------------------------------------------------------------------------------------------------------------------------------------------------------------------------------------------------------------------------------------- |

him then, too, rather than knowing exactly what is going to happen.'

*First Therapist:* 'Well, he may feel differently about it than you do. He may agree with Dad over that. I don't know—let's find out.'

*Andrew:* 'I usually see films I like several times.' [Pause]

*First Therapist:* 'You remember the first time that we suggested this task to you and you decided on going to the football match? . . . We all knew that it was not likely that it would come off, because you, Sarah, had said quite clearly and straightly that if Andrew ended up *playing* football, then it would be too difficult for you to go because you did not like standing on your own amongst a group of strangers, and we know that on that occasion Andrew did play football, and you two, therefore, did not have your outing together. This week it seems very difficult for us to look at exactly *what* would make it possible for this to work out this time.'

*Sarah:* 'I have the feeling that if I make a suggestion . . . well, I am almost scared to make one, because I do not want to be sort of thrown off balance by him disagreeing with me or something. Because my suggestions are very limited really, and they probably would not appeal to Andrew. I have said a few things but . . . but I don't like the things he likes doing.'

*First Therapist:* 'Mm. It is a struggle to close the gap, isn't it? But I think that you are perhaps underestimating your ability to be closing this gap because you came up with this suggestion about going to the cinema. You know exactly what makes it a good experience for you—that you do not want to know the plot first. On the other hand, Andrew turns to Mum to get her to confirm his argument. . . .'

*Andrew:* [Interrupting] 'Not to confirm, but to strengthen . . . my argument. Sarah probably thinks that I am just going along for the sake of it, you see. So, I was using Mum to strengthen my argument —what would you say? [turning to Mother].'

*First Therapist:* 'But it won't be more convincing to Sarah if you have to use your mother to persuade Sarah that

77

Family therapy

| | |
|---|---|
| | you really want to go out with her.' |
| *David:* | 'I am not convinced either, I know Andrew, you see.' |
| | [Laughs] |
| *First Therapist:* | 'So you have to convince Sarah.' |
| *Andrew:* | '*I* am convinced.' |
| *First Therapist:* | 'Yes, but Sarah isn't.' |
| *Andrew:* | [To First Therapist] 'Well, how can I convince her?' |
| *First Therapist:* | 'Well, how about changing chairs and getting a bit closer to her, and letting Mum out of the position of being the mediator between the two of you. I think that might be a help.' |
| | [Andrew and Sarah change chairs] |
| *Andrew:* | 'What way can I go about convincing her?' |
| *First Therapist:* | 'Well, just start and we will all try to find out if she is getting convinced.' |
| *Andrew:* | [Speaking to Sarah] 'I want to go and see this film again.' |
| *Sarah:* | 'Good. I would like to go and see the film.' |
| *Andrew:* | 'That's fine.' |
| *Sarah:* | 'When?' |
| *Andrew:* | 'Tonight? I shall be away tomorrow. . . .' |
| *David:* | [Interrupting] 'You have decided to come with me then, have you?' |
| *Andrew:* | 'Yes.' |
| *David:* | 'Well, that's nice to know.' |
| *Rita:* | [Reverting to the task] 'So tonight's the night then—don't deviate [to David].' |
| *Andrew:* | 'I don't know what time the performances are. Have you any idea? [turning to Mother]' |
| *David:* | 'I think the last one is about 7.40 or 8.10—I'm not sure. There is another quite good film on in Cardiff. . . .' |
| *Andrew:* | 'I should think it would be about 7.40.' |
| *David:* | 'The other film started at the Capitol at 8.10 but I can't remember its name.' |
| *Rita:* | [To David] 'Well, don't deviate from this. They have decided on this film and they are going out. They are going out together, and that's it.' |
| *Andrew:* | 'Yes, we have settled for this one.' |
| *David:* | 'Who is going to take them?' |
| *Rita:* | 'Well, they can take the car themselves.' |
| *David:* | 'Where are they going to park?' |
| *First Therapist:* | [To David] 'Need that be your worry, David?' |

| | |
|---|---|
| *Edward:* | 'Go in on the train.' |
| *Rita:* | 'All that is surmountable easily.' |
| *Andrew:* | 'It is *our* outing and no one else should be getting involved in it.' |
| *Rita:* | 'Exactly.' |
| *First Therapist:* | [To Andrew] 'Do you mean that, or are you saying that with your tongue in your cheek?' |
| *Andrew:* | 'No, I mean that—I mean that. I have been saying that all week.' [David laughs] |
| *Andrew:* | 'I have.' |
| *First Therapist:* | [To Sarah] 'What do you think about that, Sarah?—"It is our outing and no-one elses."' |
| *Sarah:* | 'Yes, I agree with him.' |
| *First Therapist:* | 'Because you laughed a bit when Andrew said it.' |
| *Sarah:* | 'Well, we were asked what we were going to do about the outing all the way through the week, and Andrew kept saying "It is our outing, let us decide." That was the bit I was laughing at.' |
| *First Therapist:* | 'Aha. So who decided that the outing would be to go and see the film?' |
| *Andrew:* | 'Well, it just came up just now. Since we have been in here now.' |
| *Sarah:* | 'I did not mention it during the week because I thought we might get talked out of it.' |
| *First Therapist:* | 'Yes, I see. So this idea really does just come from you two.' |
| *Andrew and Sarah together:* | 'Yes.' |

Whilst on one level Andrew and Sarah report that they have been unable to move out of the home together, yet as this extract unfolds we discover that they have been remarkably successful in preventing their parents', and in particular their father's, intrusion into their young adult world—an intrusiveness which is re-enacted during this session. By struggling together on this shared task, they seem to have gained in strength and confidence when faced with opposition or intrusion. Moreover, it seems that Rita has distanced herself a little from Sarah, so that she can stand outside the adolescent pair and assist them by confronting her husband when he feels the need to involve himself in their task. This, in turn, is a step towards an opening up of the latent conflict that resides between David and Rita, and which becomes available for work shortly after this session. Before the next session, Andrew and Sarah successfully accomplished their outing to the cinema.

## Paradoxical injunctions

A particularly interesting aspect of task work is the issuing of paradoxical injunctions by the therapist, variously described as *prescribing* the behaviour which the therapist wishes to *proscribe,* or as putting family members into a therapeutic double bind. The technique originated in individual psychotherapeutic work, and some skill is required in adapting it to the complexities of working with the family system. In its original form the technique involves using the relationship between worker and client, when it has come to have some survival value for the client in such a way that the worker can suggest and the client acquiesce in a course of behaviour even if this suggested behaviour appears to be contrary to what the client is hoping to achieve. By using a paradoxical injunction, the worker is enlisting the strength of the double bind situation and converting its effects from stricture into freedom. A simple example is as follows. The therapist asks a couple who are having violent destructive arguments to see how many times they can argue between now and the next session, indicating that he hopes that the number will be more than usual. The couple are thus put into a 'bind'. If they comply with the therapist's request, they are acknowledging that they have a large measure of control over what they previously have believed to be beyond their control and for which they have sought help. If they do not comply with the therapist's request, and their quarrelling is reduced or ceases altogether during the week, they have achieved for one week at least, the very outcome for which they are striving. Watzlawick (*et al.,* 1968, p. 241), in his excellent exposition of this technique, summarises its purpose as follows:

> [The client] is put into an untenable situation with regard to his pathology . . . . If he resists the injunction, he can do so only by *not* behaving symptomatically, which is the purpose of therapy. If in a pathogenic double bind the patient is 'damned if he does and damned if he doesn't', in a therapeutic double bind he is 'changed if he does and changed if he doesn't'.

Returning to the family therapy situation, the family therapist is frequently faced with a family system, where communication channels have become damaged by the incongruency that exists between the report and metacommunicative levels of messages sent and received. The task of the family therapist when using paradoxical injunctions is to convert the pathologically binding communication patterns within the family system into therapeutic patterns which promote change. Rather than making a direct use of his relationship with one family member (as when using paradoxical injunctions in individual work) the family therapist's primary focus must be this restructuring work undertaken *within* the total system of family + family therapist.

In the following example, the family therapist is confronted with a deeply entrenched symbiotic relationship between a mother in her early fifties, and her 21 year old daughter, Pauline. Mother and daughter have lived together all Pauline's life, and neither will leave the house, or go anywhere, except with the other. Both collude in the other's agoraphobic symptoms because of their fears of being abandoned by the other. Pauline has never worked, and despite her emotional dependency on her mother, she is fiercely critical and derogatory of her mother's subservience, and the way in which she can reduce her mother to this position. Both get involved in endless games along this dimension of control. For example, Pauline speaks quickly and confusingly so that mother cannot hear—in order to exert her control over mother. Mother refuses to say she cannot hear, because this would be admitting Pauline's control over her. The fact that mother will not admit she cannot hear makes Pauline more furious, and she therefore speaks more confusedly in order further to assert her control over mother. At the end of a session, the therapist suggests an interactional task in the form of a paradoxical injunction, to try to break into the circularity of this communication pattern. The therapist's hope is that both can abandon their power struggle over this issue and, having done so, experience what it feels like to engage in a less conflicting interchange for a short period of time.

*Therapist:* 'I'm going to suggest to you . . . and this may sound a little odd . . . but I want you to experiment with something between now and next week. I'm going to suggest that Pauline talks as quickly as she likes, and in the way she likes and . . . with her hand here [putting it over her mouth] if this is how she wants to talk . . . and walking round the room with her back to you—if she likes. And I'm going to suggest to you [speaking to mother] that you don't say when you can't hear. That when you can't hear her—you don't tell her . . . and that you, Pauline, don't change your normal way of speaking to Mum.'

*Pauline:* 'Mm.'

[Several seconds pause]

*Therapist:* 'Do you think you both understand what you are going to experiment with?'

*Pauline:* 'Yes.' [smiling]

*Therapist:* 'Let's check it out with you, Molly [to mother]. What are you going to do between now and next week—on this, this circle?'

*Mother:* 'Oh, heavens!'

*Pauline:* [Furiously to mother] 'You haven't heard any of that, have you?'

*Mother:* [Nervously] 'Yes I have.'
[Pause]

*Therapist:* [To mother] 'Just say it back to me just as I have suggested.'

*Mother:* 'Well, ur . . . well, I think one thing . . . .'

*Therapist:* [Interrupting mother] 'No, no . . . I don't mind what you think . . . I just want to hear what you've heard me say.'

*Mother:* 'Oh—I heard you say about um—you want Pauline to talk as she likes, as quickly as she likes, with her hand over her mouth if she wants to—and not to change it in any way. And I'm to carry on if I can't hear—I'm not to say if I can't hear, and, um . . . not to ask Pauline to repeat anything because of it and . . . see how it works out.'

*Therapist:* 'Mm. That's right. Mm.'

*Mother:* [Triumphantly to Pauline] 'See. So I did hear.'

*Pauline:* [Sniggers]

*Therapist:* 'I'm going to suggest that we finish at that point and have a look at how the experiment has gone when we meet next week.'

Next session (about quarter of an hour into the session)

*Therapist:* [To mother] 'What about during this last week . . . did you hear less of what she said, or more?'

*Mother:* 'Um. About, er, um, what we're supposed to have done last week?'

*Therapist:* 'No, no. About when you two were talking to each other —did you hear her better or worse?'

*Mother:* 'Oh yes.'

*Therapist:* 'Which?'

*Mother:* 'Um. Well, when she speaks slower I can hear her and I understand her better, but it's when she speaks quickly. . . .'

*Therapist:* [Interrupting] 'I know that. But *last week*—which did you do?'

*Mother:* 'Um.'

*Therapist:* 'Did you hear more of what she said or less of what she said?'

*Mother:* 'Yes, because as I say . . . .'

| | |
|---|---|
| *Therapist:* | 'Which?' |
| *Mother:* | 'Er—er—er.' |
| *Therapist:* | 'Which?' |
| *Mother:* | 'More. More.' |
| *Therapist:* | 'More?' |
| *Mother:* | 'Yes—because I think after last week, Pauline *hasn't* been gabbling away like she usually does and I don't remember saying pardon all that much when I have been talking to her. But, um—because she does speak slower at times—and of course, when she does speak slower . . .' [pause] |
| *Therapist:* | 'So last week you felt you heard more of what she said, despite the fact that my instruction to Pauline was to speak quicker?' |
| *Mother:* | 'Well, yes—she was definitely speaking slower—and clearer.' |
| *Therapist:* | 'O.K. now I want you to say it to Pauline. I want you to say to Pauline "I heard *more* of what you were saying last week than before."' |
| *Mother:* | [To Pauline] 'Yes, because you have been talking slower. And when you talk more slowly I *do* understand and I *can* hear what you're saying. But when you race on . . . that's when you land me in the soup!' |
| *Therapist:* | 'O.K. Let's turn it round. [To Pauline] Did she say pardon or didn't she last week? Did she ask you to repeat things or didn't she?' |
| *Pauline:* | 'Well, only the times I told you about when she obviously forgot.' |
| *Therapist:* | 'Mm. Mm. So . . . she some of the time asked you— um, to repeat . . . .' |
| *Pauline:* | 'Yes.' |
| *Therapist:* | 'Mm. . . . What I'm suggesting is that you both did what you *want* to do—which is to communicate with each other in some sort of happier way . . . um . . . even though the reason you did so was that you did the opposite of what I suggested. Now, if you can do it for that reason, you can do it . . . because you want to do it.' |
| | [Pause] |
| *Pauline:* | 'Pardon?' |
| | [General laughter] |
| *Therapist:* | 'Touché!' |

Thus, the circular power struggle between Pauline and her mother is broken long enough for Pauline to communicate slowly and clearly to her mother and for her mother to feel able to ask Pauline to repeat herself on the occasions when she does not hear.

These extracts from consecutive therapy sessions illustrate the prescription of a paradoxical task focused on the transactional relationship between mother and daughter. Yet its execution depends in large measure upon the triadic relationship between the two family members and the therapist and upon the system which we form. Transferentially, I fulfil a mother's role in relationship to Pauline and as such I have to be controlled, denigrated and rendered impotent. I need to try and escape from this situation, both to allow Pauline to test out and dissolve her fearful phantasies of relating to a person whom she cannot control; and also to role model for mother the possibility of becoming a little stronger in relation to Pauline. It is simply *because* my relationship with Pauline is an oppositional one, and because mother, out of her extreme fear of Pauline, has to collude in her resistance to change that this paradoxical task is a useful technique to use at this point in the treatment process. The same reasons enable the task to be effective.

## Using the format of the sessions

A further use of task work is one which is adaptable to many situations in family therapy—the changes made by the therapist during the treatment process in group composition and in the format of sessions. Professionals working with families often get involved in changing the composition of the treatment group for pragmatic reasons—and perhaps collusively in terms of a family's resistance. The absent member manoeuvre in family therapy is a well-documented example (Sonne, Speck and Jungreis, 1962). The technique to which I am referring is a planned attempt on the part of the therapist to model in the format of the sessions, the treatment goals towards which the family is striving. Thus, the format of the sessions becomes a physical enactment of an emotional reality—to return to our earlier definition of a therapeutic task. It should be said that family therapists vary considerably among themselves in whether or not they use this technique. Some, for example, only see the whole family group; others work with a sub-system for long periods of time without involving other significant members of the system. The majority, however, make use of the opportunities afforded by this technique to work at the point of the system's internal boundary and interface.

In our work with the Jones family, for example, the first six sessions included the whole family group. Our work focused chiefly on changing the dysfunctional structure of this group and in re-aligning its sub-systems. During this period, Sarah's anorexia was relieved, and while the rest of the family reverted to their concern about her eating habits whenever their anxiety level rose, she maintained her weight and became less depressed. For our second series of sessions, we chose to change this format by using some sessions to meet in two separate pairs—one therapist meeting with Sarah and Andrew each week, and the other with the marital pair, whilst the two therapists continued to meet with the whole family group at intervals. In this way, we modelled the goal of increased differentiation in terms of these basic sub-systems and further challenged the symbiotic relationships between parents and their same-sex children. By gradually scheduling the separate meetings at different times and on different days, family members had to struggle with moving into the outside world, represented by us, linked into these newly structured sub-groupings.

The use of tasks reinforces the nature of the therapeutic process and underlines the fact that it is about work and change, on the part of both family and therapist. Moreover, the use of tasks helps to ensure the continuity of the treatment process between sessions, during which time the family struggle with feelings aroused by their attempt or refusal to negotiate the task. Having assigned a task, the therapist uses the following session to 'check in' on how the family experience the task and to work with the ease or difficulty with which the family tackled it. The work of the sessions can in this way be focused, and tasks are thus a useful tool in helping the therapist to reduce the problem of diffusion—a special difficulty in family therapy, where there are so many data and so many issues and themes confronting the therapist during a session. The therapist needs continually to convert the general into the specific, to help the family to set finite goals and to define the means by which these might be achieved. In terms of the family's own need to resist change, a powerful defence lies in switching from problem to problem whenever some real inroad into the dysfunctional set is about to be made. In this way, sessions are sometimes in danger of becoming satiated in an immobilising and confusing way by the welter of material. Often the therapist needs to bear with this confusion and to make use of family members' free associations to get a deeper understanding of the shared phantasy life of the family group. However, when a more focused approach is needed, task work assists the therapist in re-defining and re-structuring the movement towards change and growth.

Like all techniques, task work needs to be employed with economy and sensitivity. It is a technique available for assisting the family therapist—it is not a method in itself by which the therapist should be ruled. Moreover, without due regard for the overall movement of the therapeutic endeavour, the use of tasks can stifle the family's own resources for healing and growth—converting responsibility for initiative and change from the family to the therapist. Optimally, there seems to be a progression in skilfully used task work. At the beginning of therapy, when the family is most dependent upon the therapist for the introduction of change initiatives, internal tasks have special value. As treatment progresses and a shift from the identified patient focus to the family group has been successfully accomplished, external tasks can be introduced. It should soon become possible for a third stage to be reached, when family members use the sessions to structure shifts and changes for themselves, and the therapist then becomes much less central in their initiation and construction.

## Notes

1 Dr Salvador Minuchin has specialised in developing techniques for working with families containing an anorectic identified patient, including the use of food during sessions. See Aponte and Hoffman (1973) and Minuchin (1974a).
2 Diagnostic simulation games are used by some therapists to re-create symptoms in the session—for example, the Ravich Interpersonal Train Game, described by Liebowitz and Black (1974).

# Chapter seven

# Action techniques

> Big advances are not made by analytical procedures but by
> direct vision. Yes, but *how*?
> Some notes for Clea (by Pursewarden) Lawrence Durrell—
> *The Alexandria Quartet*

The techniques which I want to examine in this chapter exploit the
dramatic potential of the family therapy session most fully and most
consciously. All rely upon a group being present in the interview and
whilst they are also employed in other treatment modalities, they can
be particularly effective when used in the treatment of the dysfunctional family group. By describing these techniques as 'active' I
am not of course implying that other intervention techniques are
'inactive' or lacking in potency, but simply that these particular
types of intervention often involve the use of physical movement and
include activity on the part of the body as well as the mind and the
emotions.

## Family sculpting

Family sculpting is a technique whereby the relationships between
family members are recreated in space through the formation of a
physical tableau. This *tableau vivant* symbolises the emotional
position of each member of the family in relation to the others. The
technique was devised by David Kantor and other workers at the
Boston Family Institute (Duhl, Kantor and Duhl, 1973) and has
been further developed by workers at the Family Institute, New
York, notably by Peggy Papp (Papp, Silverstein and Carter, 1973).
By using their bodies to create a three-dimensional representation of
their relationships, family members use the physical space within
the session to recreate symbolically the emotional space between
them. The therapist may introduce the technique by inviting the

family to 'try out something a bit different', emphasising that it will involve all of them. The therapist's own enthusiasm and conviction as to its potential value is an important stimulus and will usually serve to overcome family members' initial hesitation. The therapist then chooses one member to act as the sculptor, while the rest of the group becomes his human 'clay'. The invitation to sculpt can be directed to whichever member of the family the therapist feels would respond most spontaneously. He may, for example, ask the identified patient to be the sculptor, bearing in mind the capacity that this family member often has to get in touch with profound levels of family functioning. Or he may choose one of the children, who, perhaps because he is not identified by the rest of the family as 'the problem', does not participate much in the sessions and seems bored and restless with the whole proceedings (Simon, 1972). Because sculpting involves a good deal of physical activity and bodily movement during the creation of the sculpture, it can be an extremely useful means of engaging the interest of younger children, for whom non-verbal modes of expression are natural. Sculpting in fact provides a bridge between the almost entirely non-verbal play activities of the youngest members on the one hand and the mainly verbal modes of expression used by the adults. On other occasions, the therapist may choose a family member who has been silent for considerable periods of the session and who has indicated that he finds it difficult to express his feelings adequately in words. Alternatively, the therapist may decide, when working with some families, to throw out the invitation to sculpt to the whole family and to work with whichever family member cares to respond.

Having selected the sculptor, the therapist asks the rest of the group to stand up and to move into whatever position in the room that the sculptor directs. It is important that the therapist takes the responsibility initially for outlining the nature of the activity, for selecting the sculptor and for encouraging family members to move out of their seating positions so that work can begin. If the sculptor is left to handle his family alone too soon, he may get caught into a fruitless power struggle, stemming from the underlying conflicts between him and other family members, and the sculpting will never 'take off'. Having established the ground rules, however, the therapist needs to hand over to the sculptor, who then initiates the creation of the tableau. From this point on, the therapist moves in to the role of observer, commentator and interpreter. The sculptor may begin hesitantly, uncertain as to how the rest of his family will respond to his view of them. It is often important for the therapist to indicate his realisation that the group is being asked to respond to just one person's view of the family situation and that there will, of course, be others. This type of assurance usually enables the rest of the family to help to create a tableau which does not necessarily conform to their own experience of living in the family. As the sculptor proceeds, the therapist engages in an ongoing dialogue with him, encouraging him as he encounters each difficulty, asking if each person has placed himself as the sculptor intended and questioning what each gesture and position is meant to represent. The way in which the therapist conducts this dialogue will be influenced by the same sort of sensitivity concerning timing and pace as is required when using any other technique. At one stage of the treatment process, for example, the therapist might question the sculptor more searchingly than at another. Sometimes the whole of a session will be devoted to working out one family member's sculpture and the sculpture may proceed from a representation of the individual's current family who are present in the session, to a representation of his family of origin or extended family, including grandparents, aunts, cousins, etc., who begin to take on a new emotional importance to the sculptor, as he proceeds with the creation of his tableau.

The sculpture is allowed to unfold at its own pace, and the participants are then asked to share some of their feelings about the physical positions that they are in. When family members are asked to share these feelings with the sculptor, it is helpful if the therapist directs them to confine this feedback to how they are feeling at that precise moment in terms of their *physical* position. This prevents family members from lapsing back into an intellectual discussion of their relationships and often enables everyone to get more closely in touch with their underlying emotional responses to one another. Nearly always a person's comment about the comfort or discomfort of his physical position echoes the way in which the individual experiences his emotional position in the family. The words which we use to describe the feelings we experience in our relationships with others are often derived from spatial positions; closeness, unevenness, separateness, remoteness, distance. We talk about being 'put down', 'pushed out', 'brought in', or 'sent up' by others; we experience someone as 'turning their back on us' or 'meeting us half-way'. Hence, it is not difficult for the family to make connexions between the physical and the emotional positions of the individuals who are forming the tableau.

When the sculptor has finished, the therapist may ask him to find a position for himself in the sculpture either by actually putting himself into the tableau or by choosing someone or something else to represent him—for example, one of the therapists, if a co-therapy pair is working together, or a piece of furniture. Sometimes one or both therapists participate in the tableau (as was the case with the Griffiths family described later); but it is usually more straight-

89

forward if at least one of the therapists can remain entirely outside the sculpture, in the role of commentator. Sometimes it is useful to ask the sculptor to create a tableau to represent his phantasy of how his parents and older siblings related to each other before he was born. Having done so, the sculptor finds a place for himself in the tableau. This will involve participants in making significant movements to enable him to enter the group. These movements usually reveal important dimensions of the sculptor's phantasy concerning his family of origin and his place in it, and heighten his ability to retrieve significant lost memories.

The therapist needs to retain clearly in sight his overall objectives for the family at each different stage of the treatment process and to use sculpting as a tool to help to achieve them. He may, for example, ask family members to sculpt their different views of the family during his first meeting with them, instead of asking them to talk about their problems. In this way, he uses sculpting as a diagnostic procedure. In a subsequent session, he may ask family members to sculpt their *idealised* view of the family and in this way the therapist uses sculpting to elicit the family's treatment goals. At other times, he can use it to help a family member to get in touch with suppressed feelings about a deceased or otherwise physically unavailable relative. By using other members of the group to recreate the missing family member, powerful feelings are often evoked and worked through, perhaps for the first time. The therapist may use sculpting to break through a period of resistance, when no movement seems to be occurring. It can, for example, be a particularly useful way of cutting through the defensive intellectualisation of some highly verbal family groups. Finally, it can, as in the following example, be a useful tool, when the therapist just feels stuck—and desperately feels the need to try something new.

My co-therapist and I had seen the Griffiths family for several sessions. The family consisted of mother (Maggie); father (Jack); both in their 50s; the identified patient, Jane (17), who had become illegitimately pregnant and was the source of considerable anxiety to her parents; and Roger (14) who had recently been found exposing himself and who was on probation. He did not, however, seem to evoke quite the same degree of anxiety or anger in his parents as did Jane. Both Jane and Roger were adopted and the Griffiths' had no children of their own. We had found it impossible to engage Roger's interest or participation in the sessions and this time he had refused to come altogether. Jane who found it difficult to express her views about the family and the sessions tended to be dominated by Maggie. We decided to try some sculpting as a means of shifting the focus away from Jane to the family system and helping to open up other dimensions of the family's difficulties.

| | |
|---|---|
| *First Therapist:* | 'What I think would be interesting to do, would be, if you three, one after the other could show us how you see the family at this minute—by putting the people in this room, into some sort of physical postures. Let's see if I can give you an example of what I mean. Supposing, for instance, . . . um, you saw (I am going to give a 'way out' example, which I don't think fits your family because I don't want to give you ideas), . . . um, supposing you saw Mum and Dad as always rowing and hitting each other with rolling pins, and . . . um you and . . . er Roger as . . . er very afraid of them. Well you might arrange the room, by getting these two to stand up [Maggie and Jack] and, . . . um and have their hands like this, you know, hitting each other, and you might put yourself and Roger underneath them sitting on the floor, holding on tight to each other.' |
| *Jane:* | [Laughing] 'I'm going to enjoy myself.' |
| *First Therapist:* | 'That's just an example, but do you see what I mean?' |
| *Maggie:* | 'I know what you mean, yes.' |
| *First Therapist:* | 'O.K. You do it first for us Maggie. How do you see the family? [Interruption from Maggie] No don't talk about it, just show us. We'll be the four members of the family, . . . um I'll be you, Maggie.' |
| *Second Therapist:* | 'I'll be Roger.' |
| *First Therapist:* | 'Jack and Jane, O.K. Now we'll get up and you tell us where to stand.' |
| | [Pause while everyone gets to their feet] |
| *Maggie:* | 'Well, I can see you standing up straight [speaking to first therapist who is playing Maggie].' |
| *First Therapist:* | 'O.K.' |
| *Maggie:* | 'Well more like this. [Maggie screws up her face and stands rigid as though waiting to be pulled or pushed about] And Jane standing above, dangling a bar with strings on.' |
| | [To Jane] 'Alright! Come on, get up on there [pointing to a table].' |
| *Jane:* | 'Me?' |
| *First Therapist:* | 'Do it slowly. . . .' |
| *Maggie:* | 'I can see you standing up above us pulling |

| | strings. Thats how I see you.' |
|---|---|
| *Jane:* | [Looking at the table her mother is pointing out] 'No, I'm not standing up there.' |
| *First Therapist:* | [Encouraging her] 'Come on. Have a go. Are you afraid of heights?' |
| *Maggie:* | 'We feel like puppets, that's the way . . . that's how *I* feel about the family, like puppets, and she's manoeuvring us.' |
| *First Therapist:* | [To Jane] 'You're pulling strings.' |
| *Maggie:* | 'Pulling strings, yes.' |
| *Jane:* | 'Pulling strings! [Beginning to enter into her part and pretending to pull strings above her mother] |
| *Maggie:* | [To Jane] 'Yes. I can see you pulling and twisting each one of us, to suit your own ends, like a puppeteer, working us [pause] and . . . er . . . .' |
| *First Therapist:* | 'Any one more than anyone else, would you say?' |
| *Maggie:* | 'Ah, well . . . [looks around the group].' |
| *Second Therapist:* | 'This is Roger [pointing to himself].' |
| *Maggie:* | 'Ah, well . . . I can see her pulling her father. . . . And then I can see her pulling me, whenever it suits her, and then she has a little tug at Roger every now and again [quietly] pulling us all in her direction, and that's how I feel, that's how I can see the family [pause]; it's like as if we are all on strings, alright.' |

Maggie's sculpture (see Figure 7.1) is finally completed with Jane standing on the table, and the others grouped around her underneath. Maggie and Jack are both being pulled into contorted positions by Jane's 'string-pulling' and to a lesser extent, so is Roger. No one looks very comfortable and even Jane's arms start to ache quite soon from having to hold them out to pull the imaginary strings which manipulate the other family members. Next, Jane is invited to make her sculpture.

| | |
|---|---|
| *First Therapist:* | [To Jane] 'This time, I will be you. Now give yourself a couple of minutes to . . . er you know, think things out. Then put us into the positions which show the way you feel the family is for *you.*' |
| *Jane:* | 'Cor . . . [long pause].' |
| *Second Therapist (as Roger):* | 'Come on, what position are you going to put me in [to Jane who is now laughing].' |

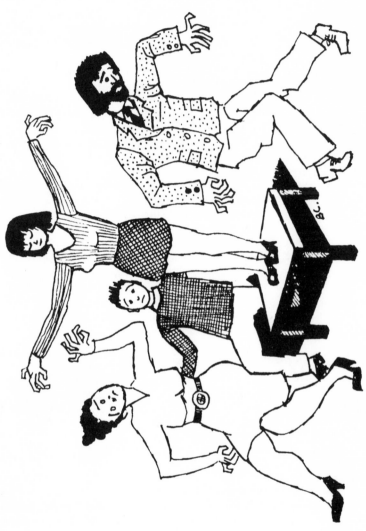

FIGURE 7.1

| | |
|---|---|
| *First Therapist:* | 'Come on, let's have some fun!' |
| *Jane:* | 'Um . . . let's see now . . . [long pause] I'm lost . . . [laugh] . . . [long pause].' |
| *First Therapist:* | 'That's a cop out!' |
| *Jane:* | 'Umm . . . [long pause] . . . [then, decisively] Right, I'm going to swop Mam and Dad around. I'll put Dad up in number one place for a change and then Mam down in number two.' |
| *Maggie:* | 'That's it, right.' |
| *Second Therapist:* | 'Did you mean swop their seats like that?' |
| *Maggie:* | 'Yes.' |
| *First Therapist:* | 'First of all let's do it how it is *now* Jane. We'll do it again how you *want* the family to be. Let's do it as you see the family now, at this moment.' |
| *Jane:* | 'I wanted Mam and Dad changed around.' |
| *First Therapist:* | 'Yes, I see, but how do you see their positions now?' |
| *Jane:* | [Pause] 'I see you as the chief [to mother] and Dad as the under chief [laughing].' |
| *First Therapist:* | 'Yes. . . .' |

Maggie and Jack take up their positions, with Maggie standing up and Jack, beside her, sitting on a chair (see Figure 7.2).

| | |
|---|---|
| *Jane:* | 'And I want it changed.' |
| *Second Therapist:* | 'Yes, but at the moment, that's how it is?' |
| *First Therapist* (*as Jane*): | 'Where are *we*?' |
| *Second Therapist:* | [To Jane] 'Where are you and Roger?' |
| *Jane:* | [Long pause] 'Um . . . where are we [laugh]. . . .' |
| *First Therapist:* | 'Take your time. Mum hasn't got varicose veins has she?' |
| *Maggie:* | 'Yes!' |
| *First Therapist:* | 'You have?' |
| *Maggie:* | 'That's how it feels—standing here like this!' |
| *Jane:* | [After long pause] 'Put Roger with Daddy.' |
| *Second Therapist* (*as Roger*): | 'Standing with him?' |
| *First Therapist:* | 'Has Dad got his foot on top of him? Is he under the chair or . . . .' |
| *Jane:* | 'No, he's just, he's just by him.' |
| *First Therapist:* | 'In a friendly way or . . . ?' |
| *Jane:* | 'Yes, friendly by him. . . .' |
| *First Therapist:* | 'Friendly by him.' |
| *Jane:* | [To First Therapist who is taking her part] 'And, |

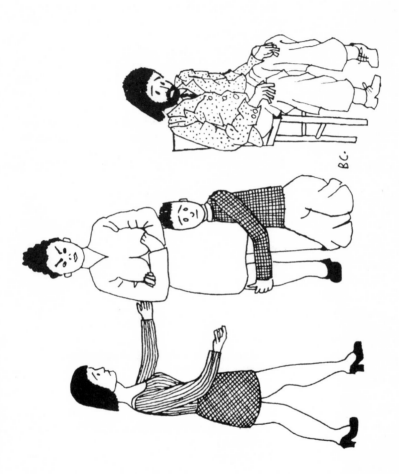

FIGURE 7.2

|  | you . . . you are by Mam, in a friendly way. You're talking about something.' |
|---|---|
| *First Therapist* (*as Jane*): | 'I see. We're close together. Am I on the same level as them?' |
| *Jane:* | 'No. She's talking to you about something in a friendly way. But you're looking up at her, 'cos she seems a lot taller.' |
| *First Therapist:* | 'Yes, and you and Dad aren't looking anywhere near each other?' |
| *Maggie:* | [To Jane] 'You are not near Dad?' |
| *Jane:* | 'No [coughing].' [Pause] |
| *Second Therapist* (*as Roger*): | 'And where do I fit in?' |
| *Jane:* | 'You . . . you are closer to Mum's feet than me, and sort of have your head in her lap, even though she's standing.' |
| *Maggie:* | 'Yes, . . . that's sort of right I think. . . .' |
| *Second Therapist* (*as Roger*): | 'So I'm also some distance from Dad, but I'm closer to Mum than you?' |
| *Jane:* | [Softly] 'Yes.' |

Jane's sculpture is completed with Maggie dominating the tableau; Roger close and clinging to her; Jane looking up to her mother and trying to 'get in'; and Jack sitting a little distance apart from the rest of the group. Next, Jack is invited to make his sculpture.

| *First Therapist:* | 'O.K. Jack. How do you see the family? I will be Roger this time.' |
|---|---|
| *Second Therapist:* | 'And I will take your part, Jack.' |
| *Jack:* | 'Well, I'll put Jane right in that corner.' |
| *Jane:* | 'Oh thank you [laughing].' [She moves over to the corner of the room] |
| *First Therapist:* | [To Jack] 'Take your time.' |
| *Jack:* | 'Well, Jane in that corner, and her mother in this corner [pointing to the opposite corner of the room].' |
| *First Therapist:* | 'Facing each other, or with their backs to each other?' |
| *Jack:* | 'No, facing each other.' |
| *Jane:* | 'Come on then, Mam [laughing].' |
| *Maggie:* | 'Right.' |
| *First Therapist* (*as Roger*): | 'And Roger? Where am I?' |
| *Jack:* | 'Bring Roger alongside his mother.' |

| | |
|---|---|
| *First Therapist*<br>(*as Roger*): | 'What, am I clinging to her?' |
| *Jack:* | 'Yes, ah, no, just stand by the side of her, and then *my* place is right in the middle of the room [beckoning to second therapist who is playing his part].' |
| *Second Therapist*<br>(*as Jack*): | 'Right in the middle?' |
| *Jack:* | 'Yes, right in the middle.' |
| *Second Therapist*<br>(*as Jack*): | [Moves into the middle of the room] 'Am I facing anybody, or . . . any particular way?' |
| *Jack:* | 'Ah, no, I'd be half and half, I'd be watching the both of them.' |
| *First Therapist:* | 'Do you mean you feel between them? Torn between them?' |
| *Jack:* | 'Torn between them, yes.' |

[The second therapist, playing Jack, stretches out his arms towards both corners of the room. See Figure 7.3.]

| | |
|---|---|
| *Maggie:* | 'He's the balance, in other words.' |
| *Second Therapist*<br>(*as Jack*): | 'It feels very uncomfortable; it doesn't feel like a balance, it feels . . . [interrupted by Maggie].' |
| *Maggie:* | 'No, I know, but ah . . . he's the centre one, that keeps it . . . [interrupted by first therapist].' |
| *First Therapist:* | 'You feel he's the balance here. . . .' |
| *Maggie:* | 'Level, umm . . . I think so.' |
| *First Therapist:* | [To second therapist] 'But being the balance is uncomfy?' |
| *Second Therapist*<br>(*as Jack*): | 'Yes, because if I've got the message right, I'm trying to keep in touch with both Maggie and Jane at the same time.' |
| *Jack:* | 'I . . . I . . . I am very disturbed that Jane and Maggie are at loggerheads all the time, and um . . . their upsetting the balance of the house, and I'm very very upset about it. Roger, I'll go along with Roger. I don't think that he, that he really upsets the house, he just rubs everybody up a little bit, but I don't think that he really upsets the balance of the family. I don't think that he particularly upsets any of us, he has his little ups and downs but that problem isn't what we are tying to get at, he's not the problem.' |

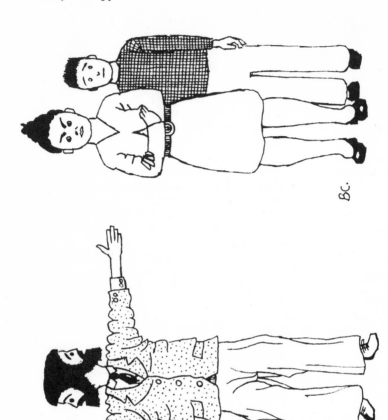

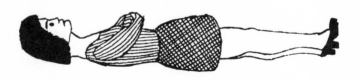

98

FIGURE 7.3

[At this point Jack is becoming upset and has got very involved in the sculpture. The first therapist decides to takes his sculpture on a bit further to look at how Jack would like things to change in the family.]

| | |
|---|---|
| *First Therapist:* | 'O.K. now Jack, let's stay with these positions we've got here. How do you want them changed? *Do* you want these positions changed?' |
| *Jack:* | 'Yes. Yes. I'd like to see Jane and my wife standing arm in arm.' |
| *First Therapist (as Roger):* | 'Umm . . . O.K. Do I get out the way? Does Roger get away from Maggie to let Jane get close?' |
| *Jack:* | 'No. Roger can stay . . . can stay where he is.' |
| *Maggie:* | 'One side of me and Jane on the other side—and Jane and me arm in arm.' |
| *Jack:* | 'Jane!' [He calls Jane over to Maggie's side] |
| *Jane:* | [Hesitantly] 'Do I . . . move over here [pointing to her mother's side]?' |
| *Jack:* | 'Yes. Now, I think we could bring it more into a bit of a balance now.' |
| *First Therapist:* | 'But *you* are way out now, aren't you [pointing to second therapist, playing Jack, who is still standing in the middle of the room, but looking much more isolated now that Jane has moved over to stand by her mother]?' |
| *Maggie:* | [To Jack] 'Still in the middle.' |
| *Jack:* | 'Well, one side of the . . . [pause] . . . well, I'd like to step along with you two.' |
| *Second Therapist (as Jack):* | 'Where should I move to then?' |
| *Jack:* | 'By Maggie's side.' |
| *First Therapist:* | 'Which side?' |
| *Jack:* | 'Ummm. . . .' |
| | '. . . Er. Well I would like to get in between the both of them and link arms.' |
| *Jane:* | 'Come on then Dad.' |
| *First Therapist:* | 'You want to get in between them then?' |
| *Jack:* | 'Between them, yeah . . . and then I think we've solved the problem, umm. . . .' |

[The second therapist, playing Jack, moves over between Maggie and Jane and spontaneously sinks his knees so that he is 'shorter' than Maggie (see Figure 7.4) remembering the sculpture which Jane had created earlier in the session.]

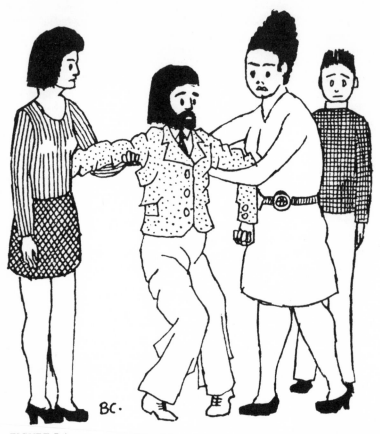

FIGURE 7.4

| | |
|---|---|
| *First Therapist:* | 'Well, yes . . . yes. Now, um, what about you and Maggie? Who's the tallest, who's standing the highest?' |
| *Jack:* | 'Um. . . .' |
| *First Therapist:* | 'Have a look.' |
| *Jack:* | [Without looking] 'I would say that Maggie would be standing the highest.' |
| *Second Therapist (as Jack):* | [Speaking to Maggie] 'I wonder if I should get down lower?' |
| *First Therapist:* | [To Jack] 'You're not looking at him, you're not looking at him.' |
| *Jack:* | [Looking at second therapist] 'No, no, you |

|  |  |
|---|---|
|  | should be just low enough to give her that little bit of authority that a mother and a wife should have in the house.' |
| *Second Therapist:* | 'I'm feeling very bent [laughter].' |
| *First Therapist:* | [To Jack] 'That's how it is. Now how do you want this changed? He's saying he feels very bent, do you want this. . . .' |
| *Jack:* | 'No, no.' |
| *First Therapist:* | 'Look, turn around and have a look at them. This is you [pointing to second therapist].' |
| *Jack:* | 'Yes, I know, I'm very bent I know, but not that much. You're not that much down.' |
| *Second Therapist:* | 'Well. . . . How's this [straightening a little]?' |
| *Jack:* | [Long pause] 'No, I don't feel that low down with her, no not that low down.' |
| *Second Therapist:* | 'How much?' |
| *First Therapist:* | [To Jack] 'You make him get it right.' |
|  | [Long pause as Jack contemplates the problem] |
| *Second Therapist* *(as Jack):* | 'You see the trouble is if I stay here much longer I'm going to have to ask . . . [interrupted by Maggie].' |
| *Maggie:* | [To second therapist] 'You're going to have backache!' |
| *Second Therapist:* | 'And I'm going to have to ask for somebody's support.' |
| *Maggie:* | 'Yes, and I'm going to have round shoulders, because I'm trying to get closer to *you*.' |
| *Jane:* | 'Come on Dad.' |
| *Jack:* | 'This, this very much reminds me of the . . . er courts in the old days, during the Inquisition, where the Judge used to sit up high and the prisoner a long way down, the idea being to make him look small.' |
| *First Therapist:* | 'Is Maggie the Judge in your house?' |
| *Jack:* | 'It doesn't . . . it isn't in that proportion.' |
| *First Therapist:* | 'That's putting it too strongly?' |
| *Jack:* | 'Yes . . . because I think that I *like* to be that little bit [pause] below the wife, myself, because, ah . . . I feel that she's got more responsibility in the house than I have.' |
| *First Therapist:* | 'But, she's saying she's feeling very round shouldered, and when we were just talking about it and sculpting it, she was saying that she wanted *you* to be number one.' |

| | |
|---|---|
| *Jack:* | 'Well, in that case I've got to find out how I'm going to be number one.' |
| *Jane:* | 'By pushing Mummy down.' |
| *Second Therapist (as Jack):* | 'But Maggie, you also said to me that you'd like to support me.' |
| *Maggie:* | 'Yes.' |
| *Second Therapist:* | 'You mean that part of you wants to be number one? There's also something in it for you?' |
| *Maggie:* | 'Well, I think a wife should support her husband shouldn't she.' |
| *Second Therapist:* | 'Yeah, but support him when he's in this kind of position?' [Sinks down again] |
| *Maggie:* | 'Oh no . . . [pause] Well, I suppose I'd like a bit of support too, you know.' |
| *First Therapist:* | 'But you're not getting it [interrupted by Maggie].' |
| *Maggie:* | [To Jack] 'Well, if you're down there, you can't support me. That's what I'm trying to say.' |
| *Second Therapist (as Jack):* | 'Right.' |
| *First Therapist:* | 'It seems to me that one of you is going to have to change. Either he's got to stay bent and you've got to get down and be round shouldered and bent too, or he's got to straighten up. Now which is the most comfy thing to do?' |
| *Maggie:* | 'Him straighten up.' |
| *Jack:* | 'I agree [laugh].' |
| *Second Therapist:* | 'Comfy for who?' |
| *Maggie:* | 'For me. I've got to look after me.' |
| *First Therapist:* | 'You've got to look after you, sure, yeah. What about you Jack? What's the most comfy for you —for you to pull her down off her pedestal or for you to climb up there?' |
| *Jack:* | 'For me to climb up there.' |
| *First Therapist:* | 'Mmmm . . . O.K. Well each of you—Maggie, Jack, Jane have agreed on an agenda for your-selves and for us, for our meetings. Let's sit down and think about it.' |

The therapist introduces the idea of sculpting briefly to the family and having got some positive response from Maggie and Jane, asks Maggie to begin. Although one of the ideas behind using sculpture at this point is to encourage Jack and Jane to express *their* views, Maggie is the most dominant figure in the family group at present.

The therapist chooses to start with her, because Jack and Jane will be more likely to get involved if Maggie does so first. During this session, family members work out their sculptures one after the other and it is not until they have all finished that the group looks at the *meaning* of the sculptures in terms of family dynamics and treatment objectives. Having seen to what extent their goals are complementary and to what extent they are in conflict, family members are in a better position to plan some of the reciprocal changes which need to be made. When Jack sculpts the changes he would like to see, the therapists intervene to prevent him from bringing about premature closure. For instance, the therapist who is taking his part, draws Jack's attention to his continuing isolation, even when Jane is moved to her mother's side and Jack's role as mediator between the two warring factions is thus removed. Again, when, in response to the therapist pointing this out, Jack moves into the group between his wife and his daughter, he is asked to consider further the all important problem of whether he or his wife is the 'taller' within their marital relationship or whether they are the same 'height'. In this way, the therapists try to elicit from the sculpture as much material as possible for future work in the sessions. On the other hand, they avoid making any interpretative statements concerning less available feeling responses, such as Jack's ambivalence *vis-à-vis* his position within the family or Jane's sadness at her distance from Jack or her covert hostility towards her mother—all of which are revealed in the sculpture. The therapists simply note these revelations and both therapists and family find ways of making use of them in subsequent sessions. The immediacy of the experiences shared by the whole group accounts for the lasting impact which family sculpting often has on what had previously been a rigidly dysfunctional family.

## Communication through action

Communication in its widest sense is the means by which behaviour is expressed and emotional responses conveyed; and it follows that much of a family therapist's work lies in enabling family members to communicate with each other, more fully and more functionally. By turning their attention to the encounter group movement and by surveying the work of gestalt psychologists, many family therapists have incorporated into their repertoire of skills, techniques derived from both these sources. Ideas have come, too, from contemporary theatre and dance, where emotions are communicated through improvised movement and touch; and many family therapists have used ideas from these sources to experiment with the therapeutic use of physical touch in their therapy sessions. The encounter between persons, which epitomises the fundamental task of family therapy, involves enabling family members to meet each other in a true 'I-Thou' relationship. Just as the dysfunctional family group engages in an endless series of stereotyped communication games in order to *maintain* its rigid system of relationships (Berne, 1968), the therapist may find it helpful to employ games therapeutically, in order to bring about change (Lewis and Streitfeld, 1970). Many of the techniques already described are designed to improve communication within the family in a broad sense; but sometimes the therapist may find it helpful to make use of a formal exercise, to achieve a specific task within the session. For example: a young couple had been coming for marital therapy over the course of several weeks, during which the husband, John, who had just graduated from university, levelled a continuous sneering attack at his wife's lack of intellectual sophistication. His wife, Janice, worked in a craft shop and was gifted artistically, but found it very difficult to express herself in words. Whenever she tried, John would cut across her with a barrage of destructive verbalisation. Janice would obviously remain at a disadvantage during the sessions (as she did in most other situations) if words continued to be used as the chief medium of communication within the therapy group. The therapist therefore suggested that the couple try to communicate with each other by using just one word at a time. To reduce further their dependency on verbal communication, the therapist also suggested that they held hands and tried to communicate what they were feeling towards each other through touch. During this encounter, which lasted about twenty minutes, both John and Janice communicated areas of sadness, deprivation and lack of fulfilment to each other. This sort of sharing had been impossible up to this point, simply because one could not speak and the other could not listen.

Sometimes it may be useful to cut out all non-verbal communication by placing family members with their backs to each other. For example: children may be overpowered by the non-verbal cues given by their parents and whilst verbally they may encourage their children to 'say what they feel', they may double bind them by non-verbally refusing them permission to speak. It may be helpful if the therapist counters this sort of manipulative ploy by disarming both sides and re-designing the rules of the game. After engaging in one dramatically different experience, family members may be encouraged to try out more straightforward ways of communicating in other situations. With other families it may be important to try to enrich their repertoire of communicational skills by giving them opportunity to experiment with non-verbal exercises. The therapist may ask couples or family groups to 'have a conversation with their eyes', and to see how much they can communicate to each other in this way. In a family where physical touch has become taboo, it may be useful for the therapist to challenge this family rule, at an appropriate point in the treatment process, by introducing a game which involves communicating by physically touching people's faces, or hands or feet. With other families, the therapist may use role-reversal, when confronted by a sub-grouping, such as mother and son, or husband and wife, who are locked in conflict. This type of strong negative pairing tends to hypnotise other members into inactivity in any small group situation—and the family group is no exception. The therapist, as an outsider, may therefore be the only person capable of initiating the rupture of the pattern. He may suggest that the pair exchange roles and play each other's parts, mother speaking as for her son and son as for his mother. Role-reversal, used in this way, can be a powerful technique for increasing mutual empathy and bringing about conflict resolution.

Techniques derived from psycho-drama are worth serious consideration by the family therapist, even though he may need to modify them in adapting them to family therapy. When a family is engrossed in discussing some recent incident in an abstract and uninvolved manner, it may be helpful if the therapist suggests that family members role-play the incident as it occurred at home. Family members are asked to orient the incident in time and space before starting the role-play. Usually everyone becomes highly involved in this sort of recreation, especially younger members of the family and, like sculpting, it can be a useful means of cutting through long verbal descriptive interchanges, which only serve to defend everyone from an emotional exchange. This type of role-play can also be used to help family members to practise a pattern of new behaviour which the therapy sessions are designed to encourage. For example: a family consisting of elderly parents and a 15 year old girl who was somewhat retarded were struggling to resolve some of their conflicts surrounding dependence and independence within the family. A difficulty which everyone experience was the way in which one member of the family would get in the way of another's efforts to become independent. Thus, Ellen, the daughter, looked forward eagerly to leaving school and working in a café, but her parents, whilst outwardly encouraging her in this ambition, covertly undermined her efforts to separate from them. During one session, the therapists suggested that the family role-played a scene in a café, in which Ellen was a waitress, mother was the proprietor and father (who was the more ambivalent parent regarding Ellen's prospective job) played the part of a dissatisfied customer. During the sequence which followed, father's hostile feelings regarding Ellen's job were ventilated through a safer channel; Ellen was able to demonstrate to both parents, her competence in dealing with both the practical and interpersonal aspects of a waitress's job; and mother and daughter were allowed to retain their interdependence in an unthreatening manner, preventing the system from being challenged too severely.

When utilising techniques derived from psycho-drama, the therapist must sense when to encourage the continuation of the dramatic event and when to halt the sequence. There can obviously be some overlap between these techniques and family sculpting, and an ingenious therapist will often marry the two, by allowing a sculpture to develop into psycho-drama, or by 'freezing' a piece of role-play into a sculpture.

The work of some of the gestalt psychologists has opened out other possibilities. Some family therapists, for example Kempler (1973), have made particular use of gestalt techniques and made a major contribution towards adapting them for use in the family therapy situation. The whole fabric of gestalt therapy has been constructed in great detail by Fritz Perls and others, and has contributed richly in its own right to some of the ideas of 'wholeness' outlined in the earlier chapters of this book. I am obviously not aiming to do justice to the theoretical framework underpinning gestalt techniques, in just one paragraph, but simply to note some of the features which can be adapted to the family therapy situation. By examining the relationship between 'figure' and 'ground', individual family members are encouraged to engage in a unique kind of situation, whereby they take the part of each facet of the interpersonal context in which they experience themselves. Thus, if a husband is complaining of the way in which a row blows up between him and his wife when he enters the house each evening, the therapist will invite him to take the situation apart and 'become' each facet of it in turn. He will be asked to become his wife, the family dog, the coat-rack in the hall, the box of chocolates that he is perhaps bringing home—and to try to re-create the part which each person and object plays within the total situation. He will be asked to re-create the dialogue and the non-verbal interaction that takes place between him and his wife, by actually speaking first his own part and then his wife's. He may be asked to change his chair each time he changes his part in the dialogue and to become both subject and object within each piece of interaction. The rest of the family are of course not merely onlookers, for they are witnessing the re-creation of a familiar and emotionally charged interactional sequence through the eyes of *one* of the participants. When one family member has re-enacted the sequence in this way, others may be asked to engage in the same exercise, after which the group examines the way in which each portrayal is either similar to or different from that of the others. On other occasions, the therapist may decide that one family member's experience re-lived in this way requires the whole session in which to develop. The rest of the family becomes a type of 'Greek chorus', participating vicariously in the protagonist's re-enactment. The family then takes part in a similar way to the participation of group members in an artificially formed gestalt group. The family member in the 'hot seat' may be asked to conclude his re-enactment by communicating with others in the room, who constitute his real family, by making some personal statement which, after his immediate experience, 'presents' himself most fully and individually to each of the other family members. If this personal statement involves him in making strongly negative statements for the first time, the therapist needs to enable family members to work through some of the pain which this involves for each of them, and to help the whole group to integrate the total experience.

## Interpretation through action

Although the acquisition of insight is not a primary goal in family therapy, most family therapists offer interpretative interventions in the course of their therapeutic work, if these are felt to be helpful in assisting behavioural change. Interpretations may take the form of verbal statements or questions and, because of the presence of the whole family, they will take on a transactional quality in terms of the whole system. However, many family therapists find that, as with other kinds of therapeutic intervention, action speaks louder than words and the family therapist can make a more potent interpretation if he combines a non-verbal action with his verbal comment. Minuchin (*et al.,* 1967, p. 248) speaking about work with low socio-economic families, makes the same point:

> In general, we have found that interpretations which employ an almost physical or 'territorial' language and which are grounded on more primitive cognitive and communicational systems seem to be more in harmony with the way in which our families communicate among themselves and therefore more likely to be effective.

Minuchin uses Bruner's classification of progressively more sophisticated modes of communication. Bruner (1964, pp. 1-2) distinguishes 'three systems of processing information by which human beings construct models of their world: through action, through imagery and through language. . . . I shall call the three modes of representation mentioned earlier enactive representation, iconic representation and symbolic representation.' Bruner goes on to point out that there is usually a progression from enactive to iconic to symbolic means of communication as the child becomes an adult, but to a greater or lesser extent, we retain all three modes. Minuchin makes use of this classification and argues that in some families, enactive communication predominates and it therefore behoves the therapist to adopt a similar style. He points out that 'the therapist can *say* something or *do* something that expresses the same meaning or preferably he can do both'. For example: during the course of a session, the children get down and play, leaving mother still sitting next to the therapist, but separated from father by two empty chairs. As the session progresses, mother begins to cry and no one in the family moves to comfort her. The therapist has the choice of interpreting this situation verbally in terms of, perhaps, the family's taboo regarding physical comfort; or suggesting that a family member move close to mother; or offering her a handkerchief himself. With the second and third of these choices, the therapist either stimulates action within the family or 'acts' the interpretation directly himself. Whichever alternative he chooses, it must be in keeping with the idiosyncratic needs of the family at that particular moment; however, a 'motor' response such as the second and third of the above alternatives, may be compelling by virtue of its very simplicity.

In chapter 4, we noted how the therapist uses the seating arrangements to pick up diagnostic clues about how the family functions. Geographic *re-arrangement* of seating positions can be used as a means of interpreting and changing a family's structure. Just as in sculpting, the therapist seeks to extract from the physical positions of family members, the metaphors which best describe their relationships, so he can move family members' seating positions within the session in such a way that their present difficulty is interpreted and the means towards its resolution is clarified. For example: a family consisting of husband, wife and teenage boy and girl, may sit so that mother is between the teenagers and next to the delinquent son, the identified patient. Father sits next to the therapist, some distance away from the rest of the family. During the session, the therapist probes into the structure of the family and finds that the seating arrangement accurately reflects relationships between family members. Mother is desperately struggling to resist her approaching middle age by identifying with her adolescent children, and in so doing, she is moving further and further away from her husband, who reflects too nearly the reality of her increasing years. The therapist may ask the wife to change seats with him, so that she sits next to her husband, and he then takes her place next to the identified patient. By this simple action, the therapist comments on several features of the family's dysfunction, and he also suggests a possible solution. The therapist's action in re-arranging seating positions in this way, usually promotes a more immediate discussion of family dynamics. He may then proceed to re-align the seating positions again and again throughout the session, whenever such movements seem to help forward the treatment goals. 'Spatial manipulation has the power of simplicity. Its graphic eloquence highlights the therapist's message' (Minuchin, 1974b).

In other situations, the therapist may make use of the technique known as 'doubling' and express both the verbal and non-verbal aspects of a family member's alter ego. For example: having watched and listened to a married couple arguing violently and unproductively, the two therapists decided to 'play back' to the couple a dimension of their interaction, by becoming the alter egos of each partner. As the female therapist demonstrated her perception of the wife, and the male therapist his perception of the husband, both were able to become more fully aware of the unproductiveness of their relationship. Sentences beginning 'I never realised before that I . . . .' are a frequent response from family members after therapists have engaged in this type of role-play. Awareness comes spontaneously; there is no need for the therapist to offer an interpretation in the more usual sense. Rather, the therapist 'recruits the patient's efforts as a co-phenomenologist to the end of *observing* rather than theorising about or labelling this act of remembering' (Naranjo, 1970).

# Chapter eight

# Co-therapy

You are you and I am I
And if by chance we find each other it's beautiful.
> Fritz Perls—*Gestalt Prayer*

Co-therapy—the simultaneous use of two or more therapists in the treatment sessions—is a therapeutic technique involving the whole skill and sensitivity of each therapist; it does not merely provide a solution to the hazardous enterprise which family therapy can sometimes appear to be to the single therapist. Although more than two therapists are sometimes used in particular circumstances such as in multiple family therapy, two therapists are normally used when working with the single family group. It is the use of two therapists in a co-therapeutic relationship to which this chapter refers.

The co-therapy relationship sometimes resembles the rich harmony of a classical symphony; at other times, the strident discords of modern music, which, while temporarily harsh on the ear, may yet stimulate creativity. The style of a pair of co-therapists may follow the pattern of a Bach fugue with each therapist unfolding his own melodic line consecutively, but always in such a way that it develops that of his partner. Or it may take the form of a strict counterpoint, in which the dual struggle of the pair involves at times the tension of opposition. Sometimes a co-therapy relationship will appear to be in the form of a solo and accompaniment, with the latter playing an important, though subsidiary, part. Occasionally, it may resemble the virtuoso performance of an unaccompanied sonata—with the co-therapist relegated to the position of awed spectator! All of these possibilities—with the exception, perhaps, of the last—can reflect a fruitful working relationship between two therapists.

It is no accident that co-therapy has, from the beginning, been an important technique in family therapy—for it introduces into the treatment situation a therapeutic *relationship* instead of simply a therapeutic *individual*. This is clearly appropriate in the context of a treatment modality whose focus is the interrelationship *between* individuals rather than the individuals themselves. The co-therapy relationship has greater significance than merely the use of two workers instead of one, for, as with the family group itself, the relationship between the workers becomes more than simply the sum of its parts. It is, in itself, a dynamic entity, which, more than the treatment interventions of either partner alone, holds the germ of growth and change for the family.

The technique of co-therapy is not exclusive to family therapy and its development preceded that of family therapy itself. It seems to have been first used in the treatment of children by Adler and his colleagues at the Vienna Child Guidance Clinic, where it was noted that some children responded more rapidly and more favourably when treated simultaneously by more than one therapist. In group work methods too, co-therapy has, for a long time, been utilised as an important means of clarifying and using the group process (Yalom, 1970). Although it is by no means universally employed amongst family therapists, it is frequently preferred by them when working with the family group as a whole. Whilst there are many ways in which a co-therapy relationship can be used—for example, for teaching and consultation (a subject which I have touched upon elsewhere, Walrond-Skinner, 1974)—this chapter will concentrate on examining the advantages and disadvantages of the technique in terms of its therapeutic effectiveness in the treatment situation.

## Creating the partnership

A smoothly working co-therapy team can only be achieved over a period of time and after the experience of working with several families. Almost inevitably, the first attempt of two therapists to work together will be ragged and uncoordinated. The two workers may come from different professional backgrounds and maybe even from different agencies. The two different professions and the different agencies may have radically different cultures, norms and attitudes which their workers will have imbibed. If the workers come from different professional backgrounds within the same agency, such as psychiatry and social work, they may also have to come to terms with the inbuilt hierarchical relationship which exists in their usual professional interchange with each other. They may have achieved differing status within their separate professions—such as a senior medical social worker and a junior hospital doctor. Whilst subscribing to the basic premises of family psychotherapy, they may have different theoretical orientations towards the treatment method, and different ideas about therapeutic style and technique. There is some evidence to show that therapeutic style is an important dimension of the co-therapy relationship. In a study conducted by Rice, Fey and Kepecs (1972) using therapists who had a considerable degree of experience with co-therapy, and others who had very little, six different styles were isolated: blank screen; paternal; transactional; authoritarian; maternal; and idiosyncratic. Therapists showed marked preferences concerning the style of their co-therapist —some definitely preferring him to have a style similar to their own; others definitely preferring their co-therapist's style to be different, though complementary.

Therapists may differ more personally and more fundamentally in terms of basic characteristics such as age and sex. A co-therapy team can be made up of two workers of the same or of the opposite sex; in either case each worker will differ in his expectations and feelings about working with the other. For example: a male worker may have an extremely rigid perception of the behaviour appropriate for his female co-therapist, which may be at variance with *her* image of both her role and function. Or, when working with a male co-therapist, another male worker may find himself blocked by his unresolved fears of a homosexual relationship. Differences in the workers' experiences in their families of origin may affect the way in which they enter into this sibling-like relationship. None of these differences on either the personal or the professional level will just evaporate. On the contrary, the moment the workers get involved with the family group they are to treat, they can be sure that the family will rapidly discover 'the Achilles' heel' in their relationship and use it to prise them apart. The two workers cannot do away with all the many points of difference which they bring to the co-therapy relationship—nor would it be at all desirable for them to attempt to do so. But in order to create a relationship which will be serviceable to the family, they must enter into an ongoing dialogue—which commences before they meet the family and continues throughout the course of treatment. It is unlikely that any two co-therapists will allow themselves sufficient time and energy to work out their relationship fully; but some work is essential. Normally, meetings need to be arranged immediately before and immediately after each session with the family. These will vary in length from a few minutes to perhaps a considerable length of time when a new phase in the treatment process needs to be planned, or when the workers are experiencing particular difficulties in their relationship. Part of this work involves the frank recognition of each other's differences. Each needs the other 'to give him permission' to be himself in the sessions. Striving for equality of participation is usually a trap if it is measured in terms of the actual amount of verbal interventions made by each. One worker's contribution may be largely of a non-verbal kind but yet be an essential ingredient of treatment. Each must feel comfortable and relaxed with the activity and passivity of the other. Apart from the pragmatic purpose of this ongoing dialogue, it has symbolic value within the treatment process as a whole; for the therapists can hardly expect family members to work openly and honestly on their difficulties within the sessions, if they find it impossible to do likewise in terms of their own co-therapy relationship.

## The choice of partner

The means by which the two co-therapists decide to work together with a particular family is important and may influence the future course of the relationship. If the team is large enough to make a fairly free choice possible, this is usually the preferred means for a co-therapy partnership to begin. Obviously, as Whitaker (1972, p. 13) points out, the choice is by no means entirely free: 'The choice of a co-therapist, like the choice of a marital partner, depends upon who is available, who is complementary to the therapist and with whom one identifies.' A therapist often has an uncanny knack of choosing a partner with whom he will be able to form a mutually satisfying working relationship—sometimes through the unconscious 'recognition' of attributes in the other's personality which will complement his own. The most important criterion of choice is that one's partner will be someone with whom one will feel comfortable in sharing and exchanging ideas, feelings and problems as these are experienced both within the treatment situation with the family and within the co-therapy relationship itself. Some therapists have experimented with working with a close relative—a marital pair for example, or a father and son team. This type of professional/personal partnership obviously entails a unique situation and brings with it its own particular problems and advantages.

Co-therapists who inject into the treatment situation a relationship which, in terms of its structure, is in reality comparable to the clients' own, wield some unique advantages. They also face special hazards. Co-therapists who are married to each other, for example, have the opportunity of providing both a marital and parental role model for the family in terms of their actual real-life relationship. This type of role model is clearly of a different order from that which can be offered by non-related co-therapists (described later in this chapter) who are able to re-model various marital and parental functions in terms of nurturing, caring and mutual trust. In addition to providing this type of modelling, married co-therapists may well be able to stimulate a greater degree of freedom in exploring the intimate sexual relationship of the marital pair, since they too share an intimate sexual relationship with each other. There is opportunity too, for the struggle towards growth and change within the therapists' actual marriage during the course of the treatment process, which can be undertaken alongside the struggle of the marital pair who are in treatment. There is, on the other hand, a far greater penalty for the co-therapists if they incorporate dysfunctional aspects of the clients' relationship into their own. Their professional/personal relationship does not finish at the end of the day for, like the relationship between the family members they are treating, it remains in being for the other twenty-three hours of the day that the family and co-therapy pair are apart.[1]

## Technique

At the outset, certain practical decisions will have to be made. Some of these will concern primarily the treatment plan for the family and will involve a discussion of the issues surrounding the engagement and maintenance of the family in treatment (see chapters 4 and 5). In addition, the co-therapists will have to decide whether they will only meet with the family when both are available, or whether one partner will hold sessions when the other is ill or on holiday. If the pair adopt the former course, they will be delivering a less ambivalent message to the family about the 'wholeness' of the treatment group of family + family therapists. On the other hand, to retain the freedom to meet singly with the family in the absence of the other may be preferable where strict continuity of treatment over an intensive period is considered to be of paramount importance. The absence of one therapist and the way in which his partner and the family group deal with this situation, can sometimes be used to gain fresh understanding of the family's problems. For example: my male co-therapist was absent for three weeks during a period when we were meeting once a week with a mother and her adult daughter. Although we had worked for several months with this family, our interest and concern for mother's absent husband and the feelings of mother and daughter concerning him had remained a totally unavailable subject during the sessions. It was only when my co-therapist returned from his holiday that I realised that, as a group, we three women had never mentioned my colleague's absence or showed any interest in either his departure or his return. It became clear that the absence of a man for this pair was too painful and damaging a subject to discuss; moreover, I had colluded with them in avoiding this theme. On my colleague's return, I shared my thoughts with the group and for the first time mother and daughter shared some of *their* rage and anger concerning the man who had abandoned them many years earlier.

When a co-therapist joins a treatment situation which has already been functioning over a period of time, quite specific and complicated dynamics seem to be involved. Usually, these circumstances arise when a therapist working on his own feels that he has reached some impasse with the family and which he hopes will be unlocked by the introduction of a co-therapist. He may therefore be experiencing a sense of failure or of desperation and he will probably welcome the potential assistance which he feels a co-therapist may be able to offer. On the other hand, he will almost certainly feel protective towards the family and towards his own working relationship with them and resent the 'intrusion' of the newcomer. The new worker, for his part, will probably feel able to be considerably tougher and more demanding of the family than his colleague. He will not yet be caught into any collusive traps set by the family—yet he will feel more secure than would be usual when starting to work because of his colleague's prior relationship with them. This more challenging attitude on the part of the second worker will in turn evoke an even more protective response on the part of the first—who may also begin to feel personally criticised by his colleague. Unless these dynamics are carefully considered at the outset, it is likely that the introduction of a co-therapist will bring with it many more problems than it solves.

The most powerful and subtle use of co-therapy as a treatment technique is the use of the relationship to internalise the problems of the family group within the co-therapy relationship itself; to work them through and ultimately to resolve them during the course of the treatment step by step alongside the family. This process obviously demands a high degree of openness, courage and trust on the part of the workers, for it involves nothing short of internalising the pain and stress of a segment of the family's own dysfunction. Sonne and Lincoln (1965, p. 183) from the Philadelphia Psychiatric Center describe the experience as follows:

> It was as if we had imbibed the family problems and embodied them as a partial element in the composition of our relationship, thus creating stress in us which demanded resolution. Out of this process taking place in the co-therapy relationship came an acting back on the family in which all messages had evidence of having been through a period of symbolic gestation in our 'marriage'. Our messages to the family, in addition to their explicit content, all bore implicit evidence of having been through the mill of the co-therapist relationship.

The process by which the family's problems are internalised within the co-therapy relationship is analogous to Jordan's idea of the transmission of feelings between individual client and caseworker, described in chapter 3. In both cases the process is unconscious on the part of both clients and workers. Sonne and Lincoln do not make clear in the above extract whether processes such as the 'imbibing' and 'embodiment' of the family's problems can take place regardless of whether or not these problems find pre-existent resonances within the co-therapy relationship. In my own experience, however, a co-therapy pair cannot internalise an area of dysfunction belonging to the family unless there already exists some echo within the reality of the co-therapy relationship itself. The following example may help to illustrate some of the interwoven aspects of this process.

When working with the Griffiths family (described in the previous chapter) my co-therapist and I spent several sessions working with the marital pair on their own, to help them to correct the imbalance in their relationship. In the extract quoted (pp. 99-102), Jack and Maggie both express their dissatisfaction with the way in which Maggie is consistently dominating, taking responsibility for decision-making in the family, whilst Jack feels under-valued and under-used. After a few sessions it became clear that this pattern was replicated in our co-therapy relationship. There was a real pre-existent basis for this imbalance in that my male colleague had worked with fewer families and felt particularly diffident at that time about his ability to be effective as a therapist. We discovered, however, that this imbalance between us was becoming more marked and more troublesome to us as we continued working with Jack and Maggie. In fact, the dysfunctional pattern within Jack and Maggie's relationship was being internalised and reproduced in ours. When this had been recognised, we were freed to struggle with our problem *alongside* Jack and Maggie, with the result that we all four began to find different and more functional ways of dealing with the division of responsibility within our different relationships.

The use of co-therapy in the treatment of family groups enables a degree of task distribution which is impossible when working as a single therapist. Each therapist can respond to different needs which family members may have at varying stages of the treatment process and each can attend to different therapeutic functions within the session. The presence of two workers—and the developing relationship between them—offers family members a greater degree of diversity and richness and enlarged opportunities to distil from the therapists' differing personalities attributes which they may need for their own support or identification. The therapists are able to divide between them the dual participant/observer function which otherwise has to be carried within the single therapist. For example: when working with a family containing a schizophrenic member, one therapist may 'enter in' to the schizophrenic's world of seemingly bizarre picture language, in a participatory way, while the other therapist observes and reflects upon the processes within the group containing his co-therapist. It may be extremely important for one of the therapists to struggle to enter the world of such a highly disturbed family member and to form a bridge between him or her and the rest of the family. But in order to do so, the assistance of a co-therapist who remains firmly outside this psychotic world becomes a necessity. It is often useful, too, to be able to distribute the therapeutic functions between two workers when small children are part of the family group. Their world and communication currency are primarily of a non-verbal nature, in contrast to that of their parents and it may therefore be helpful for one of the therapists to become involved with the children's play, whilst the other remains attentive to the adults' interactions. Both therapists need to remain in touch with the other throughout the session, continually making connexions between the two sub-groupings within the family. From the activities of the co-therapy pair, the family may begin to gain a new sense of their oneness and the complementary part which one sub-grouping holds for the other.

The third way in which the co-therapy relationship can be used is as a role model for the family. Whether or not the co-therapy team is made up of a male and a female worker or two males or two females, we have found that the two workers will carry male and female behavioural characteristics, distributed between them. Thus when either two men or two women work together, one will tend to become more maternal and nurturing within the group, whilst the other will tend to be more challenging and tough.[2] However, it is often preferable to select a heterosexual co-therapy team to work with marital pairs or families where there are significant marital difficulties or problems surrounding the shared parental function. The heterosexual team can become both a marital and parental role model for the family to use in struggling to resolve conflictual issues in both these areas. For example, a family in which the marital pair are suffering severe difficulties and yet who operate on the principle of 'not in front of the children' may be helped to make overt their undercurrent disagreements which are, notwithstanding, distressing and worrying the children, by seeing the therapists thrash out in an honest but indestructive manner some difference of opinion which *they* have. The parents may feel freed for the first time to look at their difficulties openly and relieved of the burden of keeping up a front in order to 'protect' the children. Hall and Taylor (1971) who treated a family where the identified patient, Eric, was blind, give an interesting account of the importance of the therapists (one of whom was blind) exposing their differences in front of the family. By doing so they broke through the family's defensive protectiveness of Eric's blindness and demonstrated that blind people do not have to be 'talked for', agreed with or guarded from interpersonal conflict simply because they are blind. Similarly, one therapist can often complement the intervention of the other, clarifying his colleague's comment or supporting and reinforcing his interpretation of the way in which members of the group are interacting. (For example, in their work with the Smith family, illustrated in chapter 5, the therapists, by working in this complementary way, gradually constructed a springboard from which they could enter into the difficulties within the marital relationship surrounding the giving and receiving of care[3]). The family will be able to learn from the way in which the co-therapists ask questions of each other without feeling that this reduces the self-esteem of the questioner or upsets the balance of power in the relationship. Family members may thus be helped to risk asking questions themselves of each other and 'daring not to know'. In this way, the co-therapists can hopefully model for the family the struggle towards an open, intimate and differentiated relationship.

Finally, the use of co-therapy is of direct assistance to the therapists in enabling them to cope more effectively with the many vicissitudes of the therapeutic endeavour. In a simple way, a second therapist brings another pair of ears and eyes to a situation which can seem overwhelming in the volume and complexity of the verbal and visual data it affords. Most family therapists, however finely tuned their eyes and ears have become, experience after a session the feeling of having missed a great deal of the material offered by the family. This experience can be brought home forcefully when colleagues are observing the interview and afterwards point out material which has apparently completely passed the therapist by. However, the material picked up by a co-therapist is obviously of a heightened degree of usefulness compared with that pointed out by an observer—since the co-therapist has experienced and 'felt' the therapeutic situation from the inside, as a participant. More important still, the co-therapy relationship can help each therapist to gain some understanding of both his transference and counter-transference feelings in relation to the members of the family group he is treating. Family members are likely to transfer to each therapist different images, so that each is free to help the other in distinguishing the counter-transference experience from reality. Moreover, if family members are transferring to one of the therapists a highly uncomfortable image, such as that of a 'bad mother', the therapist is helped in both his understanding and use of this transference within the group by the light which his co-therapist can throw upon these dynamics. In this situation when one's whole integrity and identity can seem to be assaulted by the strength of the family's transference, a co-therapist's support and predictability can be a life-line. Similarly, a co-therapist can assist in distinguishing from reality the therapist's own positive or negative transference feelings towards individual family members or towards the family group as a whole.

## Inherent difficulties

Despite its many advantages, the development of a satisfactory co-therapy relationship which can perform some or all of these functions is a difficult undertaking. The practice of working with a co-therapist brings with it, too, its own special problems. For many family therapists, the potential difficulties inherent within the co-therapy relationship outweigh the potential advantages, and for this reason they prefer to work alone. The family's attempt to split the team is one of the most formidable difficulties confronting the co-therapy pair. Invariably, the family will direct its positive feelings towards one therapist and its negative feelings towards the other. Usually, the selection of the therapists for each different set of feelings will depend upon the particular difficulties being experienced within the family, combined with the idiosyncratic characteristics of each therapist. Thus, a family in which mother has been labelled as being the 'trouble-maker' and source of the family's difficulties, may perceive the female therapist negatively, while relating with enthusiasm to her male colleague. Conversely, a family containing a somewhat passive husband and a forceful, dominating wife might, for different reasons select the male worker as the favoured therapist — the wife seeing in him some of the qualities her husband lacks, the husband hoping to get from him some support in dealing with his wife's hostility. This tendency on the family's part to split the co-therapy team into 'good' and 'bad' objects is a normal, almost inevitable process. It can be used constructively by the therapists in helping family members to reality test their feelings; but unless it is handled carefully, the co-therapy team can find itself becoming severely strained. The worker who is in receipt of family members' acceptance, may begin to collude with them in scapegoating his colleague. His co-therapist will then find himself pushed further and further on to the periphery of the treatment group, and will increasingly experience feelings of alienation and hostility towards his colleague. Unresolved negative feelings between the two workers may come to the surface, and the favoured therapist may use the family to punish his colleague for an unrelated grievance derived from the past. In these circumstances, it is essential for the co-therapy team to be able to call upon an outsider who can offer consultative help in examining and working through the situation.

Both therapists need to be able to re-experience the reality of their relationship with each other, outside the particular constraints imposed by the needs of the family.

The second major difficulty facing the co-therapy team is the problem of leadership. Each therapist will bring to the treatment situation his own expectations of how leadership functions will be shared within the co-therapy team. If these functions are to be discharged in a way which promotes the therapeutic task instead of merely responding to the neurotic needs of the therapists for power or for passivity, the difficulties surrounding the nature of leadership need to be discussed thoroughly at the outset of treatment. In a well-established co-therapy relationship, leadership functions are shared and complementary. However, the family will often designate one therapist as the leader and the other as his subordinate in response to its own defensive needs. For example: a family consisting of husband and wife and two teenage girls aged 13 and 15 who had been fostered by the couple since babyhood, was referred because of the behaviour problems expressed by the 15 year old, Katy. The family, and in particular mother, was extremely reluctant to regard this situation as in any way involving the family group as a whole, and felt that the obvious solution was simply to 'get Katy seen to'. The family was being treated by a male co-therapy team consisting of a psychiatrist and a social worker. It happened that both the family and the psychiatrist spoke Welsh, a language which was totally unfamiliar to the social worker. When she discovered this, mother insisted on discussing Katy's problems in Welsh so that only the psychiatrist would be able to understand. She had perceived him as the 'real' therapist, having become used to taking Katy for individual treatment to psychiatrists in other agencies. She tried hard to establish him in the leadership role by excluding his co-therapist, since this complemented her own need to remain a dominant leader within *her* group, the family, and to convert the family therapy sessions into a replica of the individual treatment situation. In this case, it was important for the whole future course of therapy that the co-therapists struggled to unlock themselves from the roles which the family had designated for them. Unless such difficulties can be resolved, the co-therapy relationship degenerates into a competition as to who can be most 'caring', most 'insightful' or most 'dynamic'; in other words, who can be the 'best therapist'! Competition can be a spur as well as an impediment; but within most co-therapy teams, especially in the early stages, rivalrous competition binds and controls the team's spontaneity and raises the anxiety level of each worker to unmanageable proportions.

A newly formed co-therapy team may encounter the opposite problem to that of the disconnectedness of splitting, scapegoating or leadership difficulties. In fact the co-therapists may be so anxious to avoid these problems that they become fused together in what Bowen (1971) would call an 'undifferentiated ego mass'. The therapists experience increasing difficulty in disagreeing with each other, however slightly, and only feel comfortable when receiving constant reassurance from each other during the sessions. Therapists experiencing this difficulty in their relationship will usually sit next to each other in the sessions and, from an observer's point of view, will seem to be huddling together against the icy blast of the family's onslaught. Just as parents can sometimes be so closely fused together that the children feel rejected and extruded from their relationship, similarly, the family group can begin to feel painfully outside the closeness and harmony of the co-therapists' relationship. A particularly disturbed or hostile family group is likely to produce this reaction temporarily within most co-therapy relationships; but if it becomes a more prolonged characteristic of a particular team, it is likely to display some of the dysfunctional features of a symbiotic tie between family members. Differences are experienced as being fearful and destructive and attempts at differentiation by either therapist are punished by the other. Within the ambience of this type of co-therapy relationship, the propensity of family members to retreat into dysfunctional and exclusive pairings will increase and the capacity for growth for all members of the treatment group will be reduced.

Finally, when considering the use of co-therapy in working with the family group, the therapists have to reckon on the added complication which their transference and counter-transference feelings *within the co-therapy relationship itself* will produce in the context of the total treatment situation. During the later phases of family treatment the therapists will almost invariably be working with primitive emotional themes surrounding sexual identity, maternal creativity and masculine potency. These themes will find their reflection within the co-therapy relationship in terms of both the real and the transferred relationship between the therapists. The way in which they are worked through will be affected both by the family group's particular pathology and the extent to which the therapists themselves can raise to consciousness their residual phantasies from similar early relationships. To the extent to which the therapists are able to deal with these primitive themes in terms of current reality, they will be freed to make use of the potential resources which the co-therapy relationship has to offer. Rubinstein and Weiner (1967, p. 215) have described the interesting phenomenon of 'double transference': 'The complicated transactional experience that presents itself in co-therapy teamwork with a family lends itself to the peculiar phenomenon of transferring the transference, using the co-therapist or the family as an intermediary.' For example, one of the therapists may experience a negative transference towards mother in the family, because she evokes for him his difficult and unresolved relationship with his own mother. However, he may *express* his feeling instead towards his co-therapist, who thus becomes the recipient of his colleague's 'transferred transference'. Similarly, a transference experienced in relation to one's co-therapist can become transferred to a member of the family group. In the face of these complications, some family therapists feel that it is preferable to 'go it alone'; however, if the channels for ongoing dialogue between the therapists remain open, and if consultative help is available, the source of the therapists' feeling responses can usually be traced and resolved.

It seems to me that in appraising the place of co-therapy as a treatment tool, three stages are passed through during the professional lives of many family therapists. First, it seems to offer a crutch to the beginner and a safe haven for the more experienced therapist confronted by a particularly difficult family. During this phase, the use of co-therapy will provide some security, but the problems inherent in its use may turn out to be unexpectedly troublesome. Next, the therapist may react to this phase, by feeling that, in order to develop his own skills more fully, he needs to work more frequently on his own. Rice, Fey and Kepecs (1972) discovered that, within their sample, therapists seemed to reach a point of 'diminishing returns' in terms of the satisfaction derived from using co-therapy. Third, the therapist may gradually begin to integrate the use of both approaches—working sometimes on his own, sometimes with a co-therapist—as the treatment situation demands. His use of co-therapy will then arise out of a more mature ability to select a treatment tool appropriate for the therapeutic situation, rather than from his own neurotic need to be 'saved' from the family. During this phase, it is likely that, although he will continue to encounter problems, his co-therapy relationships will increasingly enrich and enlarge his therapeutic potential.

## Notes

1 Personal communication from Dr A. C. R. Skynner, to whom I am indebted for some of these thoughts on the use of married co-therapy pairs.
2 For an enlarged view of the way in which co-therapists can become 'parental', see Whitaker (1967).
3 Bardill and Bevilacqua (1964). The writers describe this technique as 'counter-pointing' and identify four specific ways in which it operates (p. 280):
(1) the second worker focuses on the point made by the other worker; (2) he makes the same point as the other worker but comments on a different aspect of it; (3) he complements the other worker's confrontation by some supportive activity; (4) he redirects the discussion.

# Chapter nine

# Indications and contra-indications

I change but within a permanency.
Jean-Paul Sartre

### A general systems approach to problem-solving

Three major problems confront the practitioner in trying to formulate criteria for adopting a family psychotherapeutic approach. In the first place, general systems theory increases the complexity of the selection criteria, even while enabling the practitioner to arrive at a more sophisticated conclusion. In chapter 1, Table 1.1 analysed the relationship of family therapy to five other major treatment modalities available for use by the social worker. Table 1.2 divided family therapy into six sub-specialities, helping to refine the nature of the treatment method as it is applied in different clinical situations. If Tables 1.1. and 1.2 are studied in conjunction with one another, it will be readily appreciated that when deciding whether or not to use family therapy, the practitioner must take into account three overall considerations. First, he must make the decision to use family therapy or another treatment modality given a particular set of clinical circumstances. Second, if he selects family therapy, he must decide which sub-speciality of the method to employ. Third, having decided which sub-speciality to employ, he has to consider whether this should be undertaken alone; or in conjunction with another *sub-speciality of family therapy;* or in conjunction with another *treatment modality,* or both. (See Figure 9.1.)

This problem of increased complexity is not unique to family therapy; it confronts all who adopt a systems approach to problem-solving and decision-making. Hence Goldstein (1973, p. 110), in attempting to elaborate a unitary approach to social work method, recognises the dual part played by general systems theory in both

123

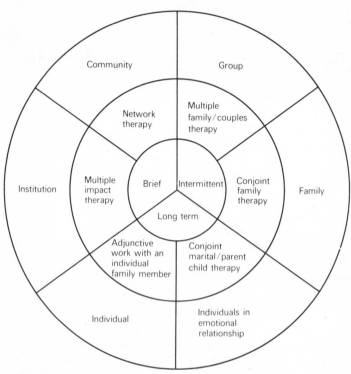

FIGURE 9.1
Figure 9.1 links treatment modalities (outer band); family therapy sub-specialities (middle band); and degrees of treatment intensity (inner band). The figure suggests the way in which a choice on each band has to be matched up with a choice on each of the other two.

increasing the problem's order of complexity and in helping towards its solution:

> a system's orientation reveals the nature of the larger social problem as well as its impact on the specific persons or groups of persons in relation. Conversely, it elucidates the systems, persons and behaviours which tend to perpetuate the problem and thereby identifies the points in the complex of systems where the most effective intervention is possible.

The family therapist is thus confronted by a multi-dimensional set of choices. Nor can these complex decisions be settled once and for all at the outset of treatment—since the dynamic, evolving character of the treatment process precludes any static solution. A decision to combine treatment modalities and/or family therapy sub-specialities will also depend upon the variable of treatment intensity. Given that other conditions are constant, the decision will be different when undertaking brief intervention, intermittent intervention (periods of treatment alternating with periods of recession) or when undertaking long-term intensive work.

## Research

The second major difficulty surrounds the paucity of reliable process and outcome studies, whereby general conclusions can be drawn regarding the effectiveness of family therapy in a controlled set of circumstances. Nor does it seem likely, according to the report of the Group for the Advancement of Psychiatry (1970), that 'widespread research on family treatment will be forthcoming' even though, in order to decide whether or not to employ any type of treatment intervention, properly documented research studies are obviously vitally necessary. The practitioner needs to know, from empirically derived and tested data, whether family therapy has been demonstrated to be effective and if so, in which situations. A study by Wells, Dilkes and Trivelli (1972) indicates the extent of the methodological problems involved in attempting to measure the results of family therapy, for these workers were only able to find eighteen studies which met minimal standards of validity. In particular, the lack of consideration given to the therapist(s) variable (in terms of his attitudes, belief system, personality and style) has special importance if one is operating within a general systems framework; for decisions regarding treatment method arise, as we have noted, out of the family + family therapist configuration. It follows that decision-making regarding the sub-speciality of the treatment method depends upon the two component parts of the therapeutic system (family + therapist) and upon the unique whole which they compose. Hence, a clearer understanding of the contribution made to treatment choice by the therapist's own personal and professional idiosyncrasies must await further research.

### Family taxonomies

The third problem confronting the family therapist is that, in contrast to individual treatment methods, there is no generally agreed upon family typology for the practitioner to use. 'The whole subject of family typology is one of the most complex, difficult and basic problems in the field, yet it is still unresolved with no clearly promising solutions in sight', comment Riskin and Faunce (1972, p. 384). Even the idea of classifying families raises some difficult questions. For example: does classification involve the construction of diagnostic categories in the medical sense? Is an attempt being made to impose a static label upon the dysfunctional family group? Is classification compatible with the concept of a dynamic systems model of the family? On the other hand the *lack* of any generally accepted typology at present makes it difficult to draw comparisons between families, when trying to assess their suitability for treatment, and further inhibits the formulation and testing of hypotheses concerning the potential effectiveness of the method. It seems to me that problems arising from the *absence* of a family typology far outweigh the philosophical difficulty of formulating a classification which allows the potential for both 'change' and 'permanency' to continue to characterise each individual family system.

Early attempts at constructing a taxonomy of families do little more than extrapolate to the family, symptomatic classifications formulated for the treatment of individuals. The identified patient's label is simply transferred to the family group as a whole, families being described as 'delinquent', 'neurotic', 'schizophrenic', etc. Apart from the obvious difficulty encountered when one family contains two or more people from different psycho-social categories, it is in any case illogical, when working from within a general systems framework, to make use of the identified patient's symptomatology to classify the whole family. Somewhat more sophisticated are classifications based on the developmental stages of the individual, derived from Freud's psycho-sexual phases for example, or from Erikson's developmental modes (1968). But again, family typologies based on these models are essentially reductive, for they involve the translation of a model developed for individual classification to the non-summated components of dyads and small groups.[1]

A third type of broad, descriptive classification has been developed by various workers. Minuchin *et al.* (1967) for example, have described families as being either enmeshed or disorganised. Similarly Jordan (1972) categorises families as either integrative or centrifugal. Warren Brodey (1967), using homeostasis as the parameter of change, suggests classifying families as 'static', 'responsive' or 'neutral', according to their ability to disrupt their equilibrium. A more detailed typology has been devised by Spitzer, Swanson and Lehr (1968) as a means of studying family reactions to the careers of psychiatric patients. Using 'propensity for action' and 'expected performance level' as differential parameters, eight family types were isolated, using a retrospective study of seventy-nine first admission patients. As a generally applicable family taxonomy, the usefulness of this study is, however, obviously limited by the particular nature of the author's task in evaluating the connexion between the identified patient's hospitalisation and his family's reactive behaviour along the two defined parameters.

126

A typology which does aspire to universal application and which isolates and describes distinctively transactional phenomena is that developed by Reiss (1971). Reiss describes a three-fold classification of family constructs: environment-sensitive families (normal), in which family members jointly perceive problems as requiring a solution by the group, each recognising the responses of the others as being concerned with resolving the external problem; inter-personal distance-sensitive families (delinquent), in which family members jointly perceive problem-solving as the means whereby each individual demonstrates his independence and competence to the others; and consensus-sensitive families (schizophrenic), in which family members jointly perceive problem-solving as the means whereby they can maintain intra-familial agreement and closeness. These three types can be compared along three parameters (problem-solving effectiveness, co-ordination and penchant for closure) to give a differential prediction of family functioning. With the exception of Wertheim's typology (to be discussed later), Reiss' inductively derived classification is one of the most promising attempts so far made. It meets the basic requirement of a family typology in that it describes families in terms of transactional phenomena. However, it is somewhat circumscribed in its applicability in so far as it is mainly concerned with the family's 'characteristic orientation to the environ-ment' and, in addition, the typology is confined to just three classes.

So far we have reviewed three major problems confronting the practitioner as he attempts to decide upon the treatment of choice for each clinical situation with which he is presented. In the absence of well-documented outcome research linked to a transactionally based taxonomy, practitioners have had to draw up their own guide-lines. The rest of this chapter will be devoted to considering these guidelines and in examining a family typology which seems to offer a means of integration.

## Indications for considering family therapy

In general we can agree with Wynne (1965, p. 294) that some form of family therapy is indicated 'for the clarification and resolution of any structural intrafamilial relationship difficulty. In using the term "relationship difficulty", I refer to problems in the transactional patterns, in the reciprocal interaction, among family members to which each person is contributing, either collusively or openly.' The following situations are presented as examples, rather than categories, since there is inevitably some overlap between them. First, clinical situations which present themselves to the therapist *transactionally* in terms of a relationship rather than in terms of an *individual's* symptomatology, almost always require family therapy as the treatment of choice. For example, a married couple may come for help because they feel unhappy and unsatisfied with their *relationship*. Sometimes a parent and child will present themselves in a similar way, feeling that things seem to be going wrong *between* them. Where family members are themselves seeing their difficulties in terms of a relationship, it would obviously be retrogressive for the therapist to offer individual treatment or group work with either or both partner separately. Moreover, their ability to perceive problems in systems terms, indicates a partly open family system which is likely to respond favourably to the growth promoting interventions of a therapist (see Figure 9.1, p. 124). Where a married couple present themselves in this way, it may be appropriate to devote a large number of the sessions to them on their own in conjoint marital therapy. However, it may also be important for the therapist to engage the children in treatment with their parents from time to time, if only to help the total family group to integrate changes that are taking place within the marriage. It is often important too, for the couple's families of origin to be engaged in the treatment process for some of the time, when husband or wife's difficulties arise from an unresolved relationship within their first family. Bearing in mind that the therapist's task is to engage the *operative family system* in treatment, it may be important, when presented with a marital difficulty, to throw the net very wide indeed, and develop the sessions towards *kin network therapy* (Speck and Attneave, 1971). The therapist should always aim to include in the sessions all persons who are emotionally significant, so that the operative family system gets worked with, not talked about, during the sessions. When the marital couple seem to be isolated from the social environment, and find the presence of the therapist highly threatening, it may be useful to work with them through a *multiple couples group,* whereby sessions are held with three or four marital pairs together (Framo, 1973). The treatment process can often be accelerated by encouraging marital pairs to work on their difficulties within this multiple group, which offers many opportunities for identification and mutual support, as well as for the facilitating assistance afforded by the therapist. Similarly, when a single-parent family presents itself, it may be helpful to consider employing *multiple family therapy* as the sub-speciality of choice (Lacqueur, 1972; Leichter and Schulman, 1974). A multiple family therapy group is usually composed of families which have certain identifying features in terms of their structure (such as single-parent families or families with adolescent children) but not too close a resemblance in terms of identifying symptomatology. In this way, intra- and inter-familial processes within the group can be facilitated by the therapist so as to maximise the growth potential of each family system, without the group becoming blocked by the resistive effects of closely identified symptoms.

The second type of clinical situation in which family therapy is indicated is where one or more family members are struggling to achieve some form of differentiation from the rest of the family. These families are usually characterised by a high degree of forced morphostasis and a limited ability to adapt and grow spontaneously. The effort to differentiate may be part of the normal developmental crisis of adolescence, which for some reason or other is creating a higher than usual level of stress within the family. Or, it may involve a marital pair who are trying to work towards separation. Or, the situation may be focused around any dyad within the family, such as mother/daughter, mother/son, father/daughter, twin brothers, etc., where the relationship has become symbiotic. Separation, if it is to be successfully accomplished, involves activity on the part of both the one who is leaving and the one who is left. Hence, the argument sometimes used that family therapy is contra-indicated when separation between family members is the goal of treatment does not seem to me to be valid. The painful process of working through the many conflicting emotions which most separations arouse, needs to be undertaken between all who are involved, just as mourning needs, if possible to begin before and continue after the loss is sustained. On the other hand, it is often extremely useful to combine two sub-specialities of family treatment when working with separation difficulties, and/or to combine some form of family therapy with another treatment modality. For example, it is usually important to see an adolescent individually in *addition* to the family therapy sessions. Where co-therapists are working together, one may undertake to see the adolescent separately. It may be helpful if the male therapist sees a boy and the female undertakes the individual sessions when the adolescent is a girl— since this further assists the young person in identifying with someone from his own sex, outside his family group. Sometimes, of course, the reverse is indicated, to enable the adolescent to practise forming a relationship with a member of the opposite sex. Similarly, when a married couple are working towards separation it may be helpful to move from conjoint to either collaborative or concurrent sessions (see Table 1.1, p. 7), or to combine both types of work. In this way, the format of the sessions models the course of progressively decreasing intimacy which the couple is struggling to achieve. Group work may be a useful adjunctive treatment modality when a child or adolescent is symbiotically tied to a parent or sibling. Rather than risk replacing the original symbiosis with a symbiotic tie to the therapist, it may be more advantageous to place the child in an artificially formed therapeutic group enabling him to experiment with some separation

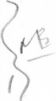

129

from his family and to develop some social skills with his peers. In each case, the family therapy sessions form the backbone of treatment, since the struggle is a reciprocal one between the one who is moving away, and those who would keep him, with mutual secondary gains involved for each member of the family system.

The third set of clinical circumstances indicating family therapy include all those situations where one or more family members are being used by others to relieve stress, which is more properly located within the system of family relationships. The identified patient may present with a wide range of symptomatology, including schizophrenia, neurotic and psychosomatic disorders and many different acting out manifestations, such as delinquency. There are a range of levels upon which families may present these types of difficulty. Some fairly well integrated family systems will present with relatively mild symptoms of individual dysfunction. For example: a family may mildly scapegoat one of the children because he challenges the system to permit him more differentiation than it is prepared to allow. Or a withdrawn child may start stealing at school and at home, as a way of getting in touch with the rest of his family, who find it difficult to show affection physically. In other families the system will display characteristics of pseudo-integration (see Table 9.1) whereby there is a high degree of forced morphostasis and a low level of consensual morphostasis in the system. A child may be battered by a mother who can find no other way of calling attention to the unhappiness she is experiencing within her marital relationship. On a more complex level, Skynner (1969b) points out that family therapy is indicated when a family is 'functioning at a basically paranoid-schizoid level, with part object relationships, lack of ego boundaries and extensive use of denial, splitting and projection'. In these situations it is useless, and even harmful, to select for treatment only the family member who seems obviously to be in pain. In one of the above examples, the operative system must include *at least* mother, baby and husband together with the transactional patterns between them which will reveal themselves during the sessions. Where one family member has paranoid phantasies about the way others in the family are feeling and acting towards him, family therapy enables the paranoid member to reality test his phantasies in the safe, containing situation of the therapy session. Families where one or more members function at this level are often extremely resistant to all types of therapeutic intervention, being closed family systems and having rigid rules controlling internal transactions. However, if these families can be successfully engaged in family therapy, this treatment modality usually holds out the most hope for a successful treatment outcome. Some therapists make use of a sub-speciality of family therapy known as *multiple*

*impact therapy* in these circumstances. The family is seen intensively over a period of two to three days, during which several therapists work with many different sub-systems as well as with the family system as a whole. Every effort is made to use the intensity of this input of therapeutic work to enable the family to continue on its own after leaving the therapists (MacGregor, 1962; *et al.,* 1964).

Whenever pathological processes within the family are interlocking, family therapy is the treatment of choice. Thus, Wynne draws attention to the necessity for using family therapy where individual family members are trading dissociations. According to Wynne (1965, p. 298), when families present in this way,

> there is an intricate network of perceptions about others and dissociations about oneself in which each person 'locates' the totality of a particular quality or feeling in another family member . . . the fixed view that each person has of the other is unconsciously exchanged for a fixed view of himself held by the other. . . . The trading of dissociations means that each person deals most focally with that in the other which the other cannot acknowledge.

As we noted in chapter 3, each family member who is caught into this process 'benefits' by not having to confront those parts of his own personality which are distasteful to him, and yet he does not have to lose touch with them completely as they become focused for him in the personality of another family member. Because of the complexity of the mutual secondary gains involved, this type of interlocking pathology makes severe demands upon any therapeutic strategy. However, because it provides an arena for reality-testing, and experimentation and new emotional experience for all participants in the interlocking process, family therapy is often the therapeutic intervention which holds out most hope of alleviating the stress sustained in these families.

Finally, family therapy can often be an effective means of helping 'hard to reach' families. Individuals who, for example, may be grossly disturbed themselves and yet would be implacably opposed to seeking help for themselves, can sometimes be prevailed upon to come to family therapy sessions, where another member of the family has been firmly and safely identified as the patient. These family members will probably maintain, during the whole course of treatment, that they are only coming on behalf of the identified patient; yet changes can sometimes be wrought within the family structure which can help them, too, to function less bizarrely. Roberts (1968) suggests that family therapy can serve a useful purpose with families who find it so difficult to resolve their 'approach/avoidance' conflict *vis-à-vis* any form of help[2] that they will only come for one session. These families are often characterised by a low level of consensual and forced morphostasis and a low degree of integration (see Table 9.1), making it difficult for their members to commit themselves to any type of prolonged course of treatment. Even though these families may never come back for further treatment, it is often possible for the therapist to mobilise sufficient latent resources within the group, due to the system being externally open, for family members to work on their problems with fresh impetus and success, without the continuing presence of a therapist.

## Contra-indications

Conditions which appear to contra-indicate the use of family therapy are even more difficult to define clearly. Lists of contra-indications often say more about the therapist's own areas of defensiveness, rather than offering an overall generalisation about the probable outcome of family therapy. Moreover, one therapist's contra-indication may be another therapist's challenge! However, there are several general observations which can be made, drawn from clinical practice. First, family therapy is obviously contra-indicated by common sense when the identified patient's family group is physically unavailable. Family members may be dead or simply have no ongoing relationship with one another to which the individual's current difficulties can be said to be reactive. These individuals may be social and emotional isolates, or the operative emotional system in which their current difficulty is embedded may have become their work or peer group rather than their family. (At this point it may be worth noting that the treatment modalities set out in Table 1.1 are more properly described as continuous rather than discrete variables, for there comes a point, for example, in the treatment of a system of peer group relationships, when it may be difficult to state with certainty whether one is employing the second sub-speciality of family therapy, i.e. individuals in an emotional relationship, or using group work as the treatment of choice.) Sometimes the total *psychological* unavailability of key family members may mean that the therapist has to abandon family therapy, either temporarily or permanently—though the effort to involve unwilling or resistant members of the family system is part of the engagement phase with most families, to some extent. Only when such efforts have proved to be abortive should the therapist look around for alternative treatment modalities, since, if the therapist's original choice of family therapy was correct, alternative treatment strategies will inevitably be 'second best'. On the other hand, persistent psychological unavailability of family members may point out the flaws in the therapist's original assessment and help him to a broader under-standing of the needs of his client in terms of a different method of therapeutic intervention.

Second, Ackerman (1966) points out that the family therapist gets involved too late to be helpful in some situations, and cites as a contra-indication, 'The presence of a malignant irreversible trend toward break-up of the family which may mean that it is too late to reverse the process of fragmentation.' In fact, so long as the therapist is not working from the basic philosophical or emotional position that his task is to help family groups stay together, his services may still be of great assistance in enabling the family group or marital pair separate from each other. But there are, of course, other situations whereby the system is characterised by low levels of forced and consensual morphostasis and with no motivation for extra-systemic intervention. These families can be described as disintegrated closed family systems. Family members have been completely overtaken by their primitive destructive impulses and there is no possibility of enabling the family even to disintegrate with dignity.

Third, some families may contain individuals who are too severely deprived emotionally to be able to share a therapist, and for whom therapy sessions with the rest of their family group will therefore only be tantalising and depressing. It is usually much more appro-priate to offer these individuals prolonged casework, in which they have the opportunity to experience a corrective or substitutory emotional relationship. If relationship difficulties in the family persist, it may be possible to start family therapy sessions after the severely emotionally deprived member has started to function more freely as a result of his relationship with a caseworker.

Fourth, some family systems sustain highly stressful interpersonal relationships over prolonged periods of time, which are nevertheless ego-syntonic to the individuals concerned. A seemingly genuine cry for help from a marital couple for example, may turn out to hide a well-entrenched sadomasochistic relationship. The therapist might struggle with the couple for years (such families are usually meticulous in keeping appointments and remaining in treatment) only to discover that he is helping to perpetuate a complementary emotional position which each partner needs in order to survive. Unless alternative means of gratification can be opened up, it is quite pointless and wasteful of precious resources for a therapist to work towards changing an emotional situation which is fulfilling primitive needs for the participants, and where there is therefore no motivation for change. In these situations, it is usually not possible to do more than alleviate the most obvious signs of distress through the medium of individual help.

Finally, there are some socio-economic and cultural situations which may temporarily or permanently contra-indicate family therapy. Whilst it is in *no* sense accurate to say that family therapy is an inappropriate treatment modality for low socio-economic families or with families which have poor verbal skills, as Salvador Minuchin and others have amply demonstrated, nevertheless it may be inappropriate to engage in family therapy if acute environmental problems are besetting the family at the point of referral. It is often simply a question of priorities. It may, for example, be much more important to encourage a family to join with others in the community, to protest about inadequate play facilities in a built up area, than to ponder on the possible connexion between a child's delinquency and the family's interpersonal relationships. It is of course very often the case that environmental deprivation and dysfunctional family relationships go hand in hand. In these situations it is important to employ two or more therapeutic modalities to attack different levels of the problem. With other families, even though there are clear indications that difficulties are arising from within the family's system of relationships, the family's cultural or religious norms may be inimicable to the philosophical basis of the treatment method. For example, an immigrant family's cultural norm may not allow the wife to express her feelings or wishes directly. In the presence of a stranger, such as the therapist, she may only be able to speak through her husband, who has the responsibility for distilling and conveying a consensus opinion to the therapist from comments made by his wife and children. However, for many therapists, even these situations will present tests of therapeutic skill in closing the gap between two differing cultural patterns, rather than contra-indications for treatment.

We are now in a better position to look at a predictive model for assessing the probable outcome of family therapy. The model has been developed by Wertheim (1973) and proposes a taxonomy of families based on the relative degree of morphostasis (consensual and forced) found in the system, and the extent to which each family type has the capacity to change and grow (i.e. display morphogenesis) in response to extra-systemic intervention. Wertheim calls this particular type of morphogenesis 'induced morphogenesis', and she uses this term to indicate the extent to which a family is likely to respond to the interventions of a therapist. Using these three dimensions, induced morphogenesis (IM); consensual morphostasis (Mc); and forced morphostasis (Mf), and a low and high value for each dimension, Wertheim isolates eight family types. Table 9.1 sets out these eight types, and analyses them in relation to their degrees of IM, Mc and Mf; the extent to which they are open or closed family systems; their capacity for integration and their predicted response to family therapy.

According to Wertheim (1973, p. 371) this taxonomy 'classifie. family systems into':

(a) two normal types (Nos. 1 and 5) each with a different social referent,
(b) two fairly integrated types (2 and 6) with relatively milder symptoms of individual dysfunction,
(c) two pseudo-integrated types (4 and 8) with more serious personality defects or dysfunction among the individual members, including severe psychotic or psychosomatic disorders, character problems, etc.,
(d) two non-integrated types (3 and 7) whose members present a wide range of symptomatology, including anti-social activity.

Whilst it is obviously impossible to fit every family into this classification, it offers a useful attempt at linking family type with prognosis, and enables the family therapist to arrive at a more objective assessment of indications and contra-indications for employing the method. Brief intervention is indicated for types 2 and 6; intermittent treatment periods for type 4 and long-term intensive work for types 3 and 8. Ultimately the decision regarding the classification of each particular family will depend upon the unique interaction between the therapist and the family; however, if an approximate decision regarding typology can be arrived at, using the broad categories proposed by Wertheim, the model offers some assistance in predicting the family's likely response to family therapy, and thus helps the practitioner in deciding whether or not to use the treatment method in each particular clinical situation.

This chapter has been concerned with discussing indications and contra-indications for using family therapy as the major treatment modality. Before leaving this topic, it is worth drawing attention to the fact that the family interview, used as a *diagnostic* tool, as distinct from a series of *treatment* sessions is often a most helpful procedure to use, whenever practical, in making a first contact with clients. Used in this way, the family interview provides a more adequate foundation from which to arrive at a decision regarding the treatment of choice. Moreover, it leaves more options open in terms of subsequent treatment procedures, for it is obviously much easier to move from the family to the individual (if individual treatment is indicated) than from the individual to the family. Even when it is clearly more appropriate to work with one or two members of the family as a caseworker, or invite a family member to join a therapeutic group, these methods are likely to be much more productive if the co-operation and interest of other family members

TABLE 9.1 Classification of family systems and their predicted response to family therapy (FT)

| Induced Morphogenesis (IM) | Consensual Morphostasis (Mc) | Forced Morphostasis (Mf) | Type | Integration of System | Predicted response to FT | | |
|---|---|---|---|---|---|---|---|
| | | | | | Accessibility | Duration | Outcome |
| High | High | Low | Open | 1 Integrated | — | — | — |
| | | High | | 2 Fairly integrated | Accessible | Short-term | Favourable |
| | Low | Low | Partly open | 3 Unintegrated | Accessible | Long-term | Variable |
| | | High | (Extra-systemically) | 4 Pseudo-integrated | Accessible | Short-/Long-term | Favourable |
| Low | High | Low | Partly open | 5 Integrated | — | — | — |
| | | High | (Intra-systemically) | 6 Fairly integrated | Resistant | Short-/Long-term | Favourable |
| | Low | Low | Closed | 7 Disintegrated | Unmotivated | Failure | Unfavourable |
| | | High | | 8 Pseudo-integrated | Resistant | Long-term | Variable |

Reprinted from: E. Wertheim, 'Family unit therapy and the science and typology of family systems', *Family Process*, vol. 12, no. 4, 1973 by permission of Dr Donald Bloch, Editor, *Family Process* and the author, Dr Eleanor Wertheim.

has been enlisted from the start. Again, family interviews may be of great assistance in furthering the effectiveness of another treatment method. For example, it may be useful, when undertaking individual work with one member of the family, to arrange an occasional meeting with the whole family to enable the individual to integrate his therapeutic work with his ongoing life at home. This is especially useful if the individual has been in receipt of individual help in hospital, or in a children's home. These uses of the family interview are clearly distinct from using family therapy as the primary treatment procedure, but they indicate other potential uses of conjoint family interviewing for workers in multi-method agencies.

## Notes

1 See, for example, that constructed by Soloman (1973).
2 An excellent discussion of the approach/avoidance conflict is offered by Miller (1959).

# Chapter ten

# Special problems

Ideas are clean. They soar in the serene supernal. I can take them out and look at them, they fit in books, they lead me down that narrow way. And in the morning they are there. Ideas are straight—

But the world is round, and a messy mortal is my friend.

Come walk with me in the mud . . . .
Hugh Prather—*Notes to Myself*

During the course of this book, family therapy has been presented as a problem-solving approach. Techniques of treatment have been described and evaluated in the light of their effectiveness. However, there exist certain emotional, technical and ethical problems inherent in the practice of the method itself which have so far not been mentioned; and whilst it would be impossible to do justice to all of these, it may be helpful to examine a few.

### Beginning family therapy

Since family therapy is a relatively new treatment method in this country, social workers with considerable experience in casework or group work may be amongst the method's students. Like our clients, we as professionals find change both stimulating and frightening at the same time. Most social workers who have been trained pre-dominantly as caseworkers view the prospect of using another method of work with ambivalence. Whilst on the cognitive level, the idea of acquiring new skills is exciting, from the emotional point of view there are usually accompanying fears. In the effort to acquire new theory and techniques, will old skills be lost?

In the very process of learning something new, it sometimes seems necessary to move to an extreme position of acceptance before old and new can be integrated. This may lead the neophyte into rejecting his old skills in order fully to absorb the new; a division of loyalty at this early stage involves too much pain. In so doing, he rejects part of himself and invites in turn a parallel rejection by colleagues who view this area of his professional development as an indictment of themselves. These difficulties surround the effort to incorporate any new skill. But, in addition, acquiring some knowledge of family therapy techniques for the first time challenges the worker's most primitive responses regarding his own internalised family introjects. More than with any other method of work, family therapy confronts the worker with the unresolved difficulties which he may experience in relation to both his family of origin and his current family. For these reasons, the worker, whilst enthusiastic, may find himself reluctant to begin. Pearlstein (1973) describes some commonly experienced defences which prevent workers from starting to use family therapy. Family therapy becomes idealised, so that the worker's fears and anxieties are increased to the level at which he becomes immobilised. 'He questions his authority and denigrates his skill', feeling that he does not have enough to offer the family from which he is making considerable demands. He feels that he has no right to expect the family to marshal sufficient resources to come together to see him as a group, and feels insecure in his selection of family therapy as the treatment of choice.

A similar lack of confidence makes it difficult for the beginning family therapist to be tough enough in making demands upon the family during the course of treatment. He may suffer from an over-eagerness to be helpful, desperately struggling to supply from his own resources the necessary motivation for work to proceed. He becomes a pivot within the session, questioning, advising, trying to 'carry' the family towards a resolution of its problems. He is as yet far from being able to say: 'Teach us to care and not to care; Teach us to sit still' (Eliot, 1930). In particular, the worker who is new to family therapy may get caught into the family's 'pseudo-mutual neutrality', whereby the family devises rules to ensure that conflict remains covert. Having managed to get the family to come into treatment, he is anxious not to upset the apple-cart by being too challenging. Yet, as Napier and Whitaker (1973) point out, 'unless he challenges the façade, everyone may die of boredom'. There is no escape from risking the probable anger with which the family will counter the therapist's attempts to promote change. Another temptation is for the therapist to try to reduce the anxiety of the session by working from a pre-arranged 'agenda'. It takes courage to risk immersion in the current affect of each unique moment; and yet to shield oneself means that 'the electricity of personal encounter is missing, the tricky tension of the here and now' (Napier and Whitaker, 1973).

Confidentiality poses a problem for many social workers using family therapy for the first time. Used to a particular boundary around the one-to-one treatment unit, the social worker may feel apprehensive about the discussion of highly charged emotional material within the comparatively open context of a family therapy session—particularly if a neighbour or distant relative forms part of the operative family system in treatment. The inclusion of young children may cause anxiety too, especially when parents express the fear that 'everything we say will go straight back to Johnnie's teacher'. More complicated still are the issues of confidentiality which surround the running of a multiple couples or multiple family group. The therapist may hold unacknowledged fears that severe difficulties shared in the group by one family may somehow 'contaminate' less dysfunctional families or that the open sharing of sexual phantasies *vis-à-vis* other members of a multiple couples group, may lead to a general exchange of marital partners! Again, tricky ethical and legal problems surround the use of audio-visual recording equipment. Can a reasonable balance be achieved between safeguarding the family's right to privacy, whilst enabling the therapist to allow his colleagues reasonable access to his clinical material for the purpose of offering him assistance and criticism? (Most therapists ask all family members to sign a form, giving their consent to the sharing of audio-visual material with professional colleagues at the therapist's discretion (Rosenbaum, 1970).) The family therapist needs first to be sure of his own feelings on this difficult issue, and then to take time to deal with the family's anxieties regarding the confidentiality of the sessions. Usually, the family + therapist configuration can find a mutually comfortable solution, so long as the difficulty is faced and shared openly in the sessions and not allowed to remain covert and unacknowledged.

Many of the initial difficulties can be overcome if the social worker who is using family therapy for the first time has some congenial support group within his agency to whom he can turn. It is usually possible to interest colleagues and senior staff in new ways of working if their co-operation is enlisted from the start. In addition, it is often possible to get informal assistance and encouragement from interested persons in other agencies where family therapy is being practised as a regular method of intervention. (A brief list of some of these agencies is given in the Appendix.) Sometimes a co-therapy team can be formed between workers in two agencies, so that early feelings of apprehension are shared. Working as a 'loner' without a support group to which one can bring one's doubts and difficulties is usually unproductive and costly in terms of emotional expenditure, especially when, according to the therapist's perception, his therapeutic work does not seem to be helpful to the families with which he is working. (Some preliminary research conducted at the Family Institute, Cardiff, has shown that in a comparative study of therapists' and families' perceptions of change and treatment outcome, the therapists' perceptions are consistently more pessimistic than those of the families.) Because of the high degree of emotional involvement demanded in family therapy and because of the complexity of some of the problems which the therapist is likely to face, supervisory help from peers or seniors is a necessity for most of us and should be sought from the outset by workers making use of this method for the first time.

## The inclusion of young children in the treatment sessions

If one was to ask the next person one met who he would include as being members of his family, he would be unlikely to say, 'everyone over the age of eight, who can express himself adequately in words'. Yet, surprisingly, many family therapists use this sort of criterion in drawing their boundary around the treatment group (for example, Bell, 1961). As a result, toddlers and babies are often not included in the sessions. This seems a particularly illogical means of deciding upon the group's boundary, and whilst it may be understandable in terms of the practical problems involved, it is hard to defend in terms of systems theory. The inclusion of young children does, however, pose the therapist with undeniable problems. In the first instance, the presence of toddlers can quickly raise the level of noise and chaos to beyond the limit which the therapist feels is tolerable. He may become anxious that the real 'work' is being inhibited and he may experience the parents' disapproval that 'nothing seems to be getting done in the sessions'. Second, the therapist may feel it to be too complex a task in terms of the skill and attention required, to undertake the job of 'translation' between the adult world of abstract concepts and verbal communication and the young child's world of non-verbal expression and concrete imagery. Yet it may be just this welding together of the two polarised experiences which the family needs in order to reintegrate the split off aspects of their interpersonal life. For example: in a family which is experiencing difficulties around giving and taking from each other, it may be the toddler who shows how this can be done by giving and 'asking for' toys in a direct and spontaneous way. It is usually the youngest members of the family who are uninhibited enough to express their moment by moment feelings of fear, joy, pain or happiness during the course of the session, and in so doing, they act as an important barometer of the current affect in the whole group. Even the youngest baby is capable of picking up and expressing the moments of tension which his mother is experiencing but not revealing. In moments of great distress, it may only be the toddler who is capable of giving comfort to his more inhibited parents and siblings.

Third, the therapist may, on an unconscious level, be reluctant to get too close again to the child in himself which he both envies and fears. The presence of young children in the context of the family of which they are part, may re-arouse feelings of longing in the therapist; as Zilbach, Bergel and Gass (1972, p. 388) point out, 'therapists have had to renounce the world of childhood with varying degrees of reluctance; the danger of having those feelings re-aroused is not to be discounted'.

Fourth, the difficulty of relating appropriately to a group of family members, where there is such enormous disparity in their ages and interests, can be daunting. No therapist working with an artificial treatment group would be confronted with such an ill-matched and ill-selected group of clients as the family group presents. The therapist is faced with having to respond appropriately —in terms of his language, demeanour and non-verbal interaction— to adults and children in quick succession. This involves paying equal respect and attention to the contributions made by each child, respecting him as a person in his own right, with his own unique areas of need (Satir, 1964). At the same time, he must be careful neither to undermine nor replace the parents' authority in relation to their children. Children of all ages can manipulate the therapeutic occasion to win a battle in the ongoing war with their parents over bed time, pocket money, etc., and the therapist must be alert to this sort of manoeuvre.

Finally the therapist may be inhibited by his feelings of protectiveness towards young children. He may feel anxious when sexual material begins to be discussed or when latent conflict between the parents erupts into violence. Whilst there will obviously be times when it is absolutely appropriate to schedule a series of marital sessions within the overall treatment programme, it is important for the therapist to try to be sure that the decision to exclude the children is a response to the therapeutic needs of the family and not to his own unconscious fears as therapist. It is appropriate to model privacy in the format of the sessions, where family members can deal with areas of their life which are rightly private within the family as a whole; but it is important to avoid colluding in the family's pathological defence of 'secrecy' whereby anxiety provoking material is forced to remain beyond the reach of the therapy sessions. Jones and Dowling (1974) have pointed out how the therapist often reveals himself in this matter of privacy by his reluctance to provide private sessions for young children to receive help in dealing with *their* powerful sexual phantasies. Whilst the parents' right to privacy regarding their intimate sex life is usually acknowledged, there is seldom a corresponding respect for the important private material generated by the youngest family members. The therapist may feel reluctant to include young children in the sessions because he feels protective towards the *parents*. He may feel that they are not capable of sharing the session with the constant demands which the children impose. He may also be anxious that the children's spontaneity will reveal, too quickly, dysfunctional areas of family relationships. The pace of change set by the children is often too fast for the parents, and the therapist has to perform a tricky balancing act between protecting the parents' defences without inhibiting the children's change-promoting interventions.

Despite these difficulties, the youngest members of the family have a right to be included in family therapy sessions. If the family is dysfunctional, then the smallest child will be affected to a greater or lesser extent, and the therapist's most important achievement may be prophylactic in relation to the youngest members. It behoves him therefore to maximise the potential of these important members of the treatment group. To do this, the therapist will need to organise the room in which he sees the family in such a way that it is welcoming and interesting for the youngest members. If the family is large, and there are several small children, it may be important to hold the sessions at home rather than in the office; but it is often useful to have some of the work done on the therapist's territory especially when video-taping facilities are available to record the rich non-verbal content generated by the children's communicational processes. The way in which the children react to the therapist's territory will provide many clues about the way in which the family relates to the outside world. They will not yet have acquired the 'social graces' which may inhibit their parents' spontaneous reactions (Ackerman, 1970a).

Play material is an important aid and allows children both to express their feelings non-verbally and to retreat from the session if it becomes too anxiety provoking for them. Unstructured toys such as plasticine and drawing materials allow children to express themselves most freely. Toys are not given simply to occupy the children or keep them quiet but in order to give them an age-appropriate communicational channel, and the therapist's task is to promote an ongoing translation between the child and adult modes of expression. When a child has completed a drawing, it is important that the group as a whole try to ponder upon what it might mean in terms of the family's current struggle. For example, while his parents were discussing his removal to a children's home during a first interview, a little boy was drawing a picture of a bird flying off the page in an otherwise empty drawing. At the end of treatment he was drawing pictures of houses, filled with two parents and a little boy. In another family, where a small girl was being battered by her mother, the child made clay models of two mothers —one a soft comfortable looking mother duck (her hope for the future) and the other, a witch (her fear of the present). Apart from her play activities, this child never spoke during the sessions, and her drawings and models were her only means of communicating her feelings.

In situations where the problem is presented as a transactional difficulty between parents and children, the children's presence is obviously indispensable. When parents seem unable to control a destructive 4 year old, the therapist can role-model for the family a balanced response restraining the child's destructive aggression but confirming his need to express his angry feelings. Parents may lack confidence in asserting their own needs and both parent and child may be enormously relieved when the therapist physically restrains the child's temper tantrum. By providing structure around the expression of fearful or aggressive feelings, young children can feel comforted that their phantasies of omnipotent destructiveness can be controlled. Likewise, by seeing their parents fight openly, in the safe, containing atmosphere of the therapy session, children can be re-assured that the fights they see at home need not destroy either their parents or themselves, and that in the therapy sessions, healing and change can begin.

Special problems may surround the inclusion of children in the session, when they are fostered or adopted[1] or where there is a step-parent. Sometimes there are several 'parental' figures in families which form part of a commune, and it may be desirable to treat the situation via a multiple family group if other members of the commune are willing. When it is the parents' second marriage, and where each partner brings children from his or her first marriage, the 'joint' child of the current relationship often wields special power. Problems of sharing are often severe, and the whole family, including the older children, may put pressure on the therapist to exclude the new baby belonging to both marital partners. Yet this new baby symbolises both the difficulties and the potential of the newly formed family unit, and it is therefore especially important that he or she is brought to the sessions. Family therapy can be a particularly effective means of working with families where some or all of the children are either fostered or adopted. Yet these families may have special difficulty in asking for help. Both parents and children fear the criticism they imagine will come if they draw attention to their difficulties. Moreover, foster and adoptive parents have often become accustomed to 'talking about' their difficulties in the absence of the children during the regular visits of social workers. These situations demand particular skill on the therapist's part during the engagement phase, if the family is to be enabled to share their well hidden areas of dysfunction openly with each other and with the therapist during the treatment sessions.

## Records

In any form of group therapy, record-keeping poses special problems. It is difficult to find an appropriate method of organising the volume and complexity of the data which each session generates in such a way that the data can be recorded meaningfully. The same difficulty occurs in family therapy, when the therapist has to struggle with observing, remembering and then writing up the changes which are taking place in terms of the family's structure and the ways in which each individual member of the group, including himself, is responding. A tape recorder is obviously a useful *aide-mémoire* but it does not help the therapist in his difficult task of summarising and synthesising the chief emotional events of each session.

It is normally quite pointless to attempt some form of moment by moment description of the content of the session, such as a process record. If a complete account of the content of the session is needed for a particular purpose (for research, for example) the session can be tape recorded and typed up verbatim afterwards. More usually, records are required by the therapist, to assist him in focusing his therapeutic work; and by the agency for whom he works. If family therapy is being introduced into a generic, multi-method agency for the first time, it may be necessary to adapt the usual forms to allow the worker to record his family therapy sessions in a way which helps rather than hinders his therapeutic work. It may, for example, be impossible for him to complete the usual history-taking application form on each family member at the outset of treatment, if he is trying to work from within an ahistorical frame of reference.

Because the needs of each worker and each agency situation are different, it would be impossible to draw up a blueprint for recording family therapy sessions. However, some ideas may be helpful, which the reader can adapt to his own work situation. It is usually a good idea to record the *theme* of each session. Even though there is tremendous variety in terms of subject matter in a series of sessions with the same family, there is usually some thematic continuity. It might be appropriate to record the theme simply in one word such as 'depression'; 'frustration'; 'weight'; 'movement'; or it may be more useful to write two or three sentences about one's overall impression of how the session seemed to be. It is important to record one's own *feelings* about the session, as soon as possible, since no audio-visual aid, however useful in other respects, can record the inner emotional responses of any of the group members. Thus a record of the therapist's own feeling responses provides a reflection of the session's mood and affect, to which it may be useful to refer on a subsequent occasion. Just as first impressions of the family have particular value, the therapist's reactions immediately after the session have a special freshness and relevance, which it is usually impossible to capture a few days, or even hours later. In family therapy, some notes written in the moments immediately after a session are much more valuable therapeutically than a detailed 'objective' report written later.

Diagrammatic methods of recording are particularly useful in family therapy, because they enable the therapist to capture complicated non-verbal interaction in a simple way. It is always useful to record the seating arrangements and any changes that occurred in these during the course of the session. A simple diagram can be constructed of each member's seating position and, if this is put at the beginning of each report, changes of considerable importance within the family system can often be seen at a glance. Sociograms are useful means of recording the overall affective interaction of a session. Sometimes it is possible to construct two or more sociograms of one session, if there have been dramatic shifts in the patterns of interrelationships during the course of the session. The sociogram can be adapted to record whatever the therapist feels is most important, and by devising a simple 'key', several different levels of interaction can be recorded within one diagram. Cox (1973) describes a particularly useful diagrammatic recording tool—the interaction chronogram—devised to record group therapy sessions, but easily adaptable to family therapy. Cox (1974) describes the chronogram as 'a heuristic device for rapidly recording sequential group therapy sessions'. The chronogram (see Figure 10.1) consists of a circular arrangement of 'dials', each 'dial' representing a member of the treatment group, including the therapist(s). Each dial is divided into three parts depicting the beginning, middle and end phases of the session.

The way the dial is divided allows the therapist to record each family member's significant interventions at each particular phase of the session. This obviously makes the chronogram especially useful, as the significance of an individual's intervention differs according to which phase of the session it takes place in. For example, if father has sat silent throughout the whole session almost anything he says during the last few minutes is of importance; whilst the same comment or non-verbal intervention might be immaterial if

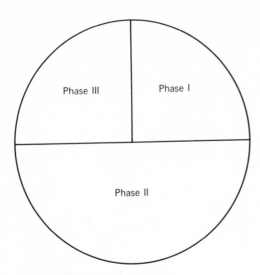

FIGURE 10.1 *The chronogram*

made in the midst of a continuous flow of verbal activity during the middle phase of the session. When the individual dials are arranged in a circle (or other shape, if that more accurately records how people were sitting), interactive phenomena can also be recorded by treating the dials as end points of a sociogram. Each dial should be labelled with the family member's or therapist's name. Figure 10.2 gives an example of the way the chronogram can be used. It will be noted that the space afforded by the dials of the chronogram precludes any lengthy description of events or processes. It provides instead a method of noting down the salient transactional events that occur during the session.

## The problem of power

The concept of power is an aspect of the therapeutic relationship which contains within it a paradox; it signifies the capacity for both potency and for control. Even when power is understood as meaning simply potency, it is still a quality which is both sought after and feared in any helping person. But what of those aspects of therapeutic power which can be expressed in manipulative control over other people's lives? Can potency—the power to assist in bringing about change—exist without manipulation? Is it possible (and permissible) to manipulate the family towards its own treatment goals, without at the same time violating its freedom and integrity? On the other hand, is non-manipulative therapy (of any kind) an illusion?

147

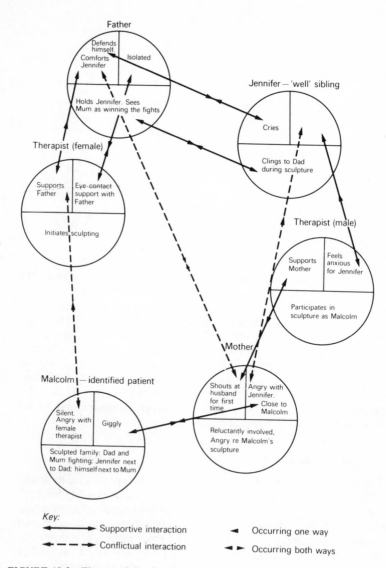

**Father**

- Defends himself. Comforts Jennifer
- Isolated
- Holds Jennifer. Sees Mum as winning the fights

**Jennifer — 'well' sibling**

- Cries
- Clings to Dad during sculpture

**Therapist (female)**

- Supports Father
- Eye-contact support with Father
- Initiates sculpting

**Therapist (male)**

- Supports Mother
- Feels anxious for Jennifer
- Participates in sculpture as Malcolm

**Mother**

- Shouts at husband for first time
- Angry with Jennifer. Close to Malcolm
- Reluctantly involved. Angry re Malcolm's sculpture

**Malcolm — identified patient**

- Silent. Angry with female therapist
- Giggly
- Sculpted family: Dad and Mum fighting; Jennifer next to Dad; himself next to Mum

Key:

➤ Supportive interaction    ◄ Occurring one way

◄--► Conflictual interaction    ◄► Occurring both ways

FIGURE 10.2  *The use of the chronogram*

Jordan (1972) criticises the manipulative quality which he discerns in family therapy, even in the diagnostic stage, during which the therapist tries to get the focus shifted away from the identified patient to the family system as a whole. Comparing 'American' family therapy with 'British' family casework, Jordan remarks (p. 12):

> people who approach an agency in this country [have] the advantage (which perhaps they deserve) of being able to present their social problems in their own terms. It takes away from the worker the power to re-define the problem completely in his terms.

By inference, we can assume that Jordan perceives the family therapist as having this power. Others have perceived in family therapists a readiness to be more directive in promoting change in the therapeutic system, than therapists using other types of psycho-social treatment procedures. Does this mean that family therapy permits the therapist to indulge the exhibitionist and megalomaniac tendencies which lurk in us all? What sort of a god-like figure is the family therapist who has the power to make and break families and to indulge his own half-conscious need to wipe out his 'loathed childhood and all that remains of it' (Sartre, 1964) by creating the perfect family unit for his clients? What kind of voyeuristic needs does he satisfy by living vicariously within the families of others? This phantasied power of the family therapist holds both a fear and a fascination, and here it is only possible to raise questions rather than provide solutions to some of these underlying anxieties.

Inevitably we all become involved in our particular area of the 'helping professions' with a mixture of motives and with an ever changing balance sheet which moves between the more and the less acceptable of these—for there is no qualitative difference between the emotional struggle of the therapist and that of the family he treats. The question at issue is surely not whether family therapy is manipulative, but whether it involves a significantly different degree of manipulation or invites a gross misuse of therapeutic authority, compared with other treatment methods. The phantasy portrays a weak and vulnerable family group, cowering before the onslaught of an omniscient and omnipotent therapist. Yet common sense informs us that the caseworker or psycho-analyst in his secluded world of one-to-one intervention has a much more uneven balance of power tipped in his favour. The passive power of the analytic couch, the subtle manipulation of the casework situation, contrast markedly with the vulnerability of the family therapist. The power of the 'psychotherapeutic ideology' is described by North (1972, p. 25) as a combination of myth and sobriety that embodies the hopes and fantasies of people living in a disenchanted world in which the very rationality and scientific method that achieved disenchantment have paradoxically re-enchanted great areas of it again. It presents itself as a science and as a technique of rational control but it is actually a form of inverted transcendence, a neo-mysticism in which the 'real self' is discoverable not by an ascent to heaven but by a descent into the depths with a guide.

In whatever way the 'real self' is discovered in individual treatment, the myth of the psychotherapeutic ideology holds within it the power of primitive imaginings, and the individual therapist partakes of the powerfulness of the myth that underscores the method in the perceptions of his clients. Since the research undertaken by Truax and Carkhuff (1967), none of us can dismiss the sobering possibility that, far from being ineffective, the therapist's influence can actually be psychonoxious in relation to those he is trying to help. Lidz (1974, p. xv) has drawn attention to the same possibility in family therapy:

> The inexperienced therapist can inadvertently promote disorganisation of an individual or of a family because of his countertransference to a family member, his transference of his own family problems into the situation, his exasperation with the rigidities or lack of empathy of family members, his shock at the cruelties that may go on within a family, his narcissistic needs, or simply by lack of recognition of his own limitations, as well as in still other ways

and he recognises that,

> any form of therapy that can promote significant change in the individual or family can also misfire and cause harm.

Even so, for the family therapist, the one-to-one situation seems to afford none of the checks and balances built into family therapy. The re-definition of the family's problems, of which Jordan complains, emerges not from the therapist alone but from the newly formed therapeutic system of family + family therapist. Just as family therapy is able to assist in the redistribution of power within the politics of the family, via the workings of the therapeutic system, it is also able to check tendencies on the part of the therapist to misuse his position. Re-alignments within the family and within the co-therapy relationship can be used to check the therapist in a way which is impossible when the single client relates to the single therapist in a dyadic situation. It *is* possible for any helping person to use the authority which comes from being a therapist to gratify his own neurotic needs. But this possibility seems more remote in the family therapy situation than when working as a caseworker, or even with an artificially formed therapeutic group.

The negative connotation of the manipulative aspect of therapeutic power has been stressed, because this is how it is usually perceived. However, many of the techniques described in this book illustrate the way in which the therapist can use manipulation therapeutically, to enable the family to move nearer to its treatment goals. Haley (1963) has drawn attention to this central paradox of psycho-social treatment by pointing out how all treatment interventions involve manipulating the client towards a position from which he is *less* able to be manipulated by conflict from within or by pressure from without. As Jackson (1963, p. viii) points out, 'therapy becomes manipulative, in the opprobrious sense of the term, only when the therapist is using the patient for various covert financial and/or power reasons that have little to do with the patient's best interests'. By a continual humble attention to his own deficiencies the family therapist, like other helping persons, must hope that within the constraints of the family + therapist configuration, his interventions will usually tend towards promoting the family's 'best interests'.

## The family therapist's ideology

Whatever skills or techniques the family therapist may acquire, his personal style and value system will be the most important factors influencing his therapeutic work, for a family therapist is for Kempler (1975) a 'human being skilful, not a skilful human being'. The therapist's own ideology will underpin all his thought and action as a therapist. His approach to families will depend as much on his personal view of the central issues of life—sexuality, love, suffering and death—as it will on his techniques and theoretical framework. For the family potentially embodies the whole spectrum of human experience. In particular, we might say that the family therapist needs to have a particular relationship with his own pain, whereby he carries within himself an ever-present awareness of what human suffering and the many little deaths of daily life mean to him.

Moreover, personal ideology as well as theoretical formulations will contribute to the family therapist's view of the relationship between whole and part, which is such a vital element in his therapeutic work. Social psychologists have criticised the way in which family therapists tend to dissolve the distinction between the individual and the family group so that the two become 'merged and obscured'. Pearson (1974) for example, views the family therapist's reliance upon systems theory as tending to negate the nature of the moral commitment which is involved in the individual's choice to be part of, or parted from, a family group, and he calls for a 'humanised conception of the family'. Viewed from the vantage point of the behavioural scientist, the family therapist's conception of the person and the group as being 'dual aspects of a single process' should not lead him to view this duality as a mere artifact 'separable only for the convenience of verbal description' (Ransom, 1972). The identity of the part is not subsumed within the whole; but the complementarity and essential interrelationship of each is postulated as the fundamental axiom of therapeutic intervention. For Kempler (1975, penultimate page), 'A family has as its sole purpose the task of creating individuals . . . . Individual differentiation without loss of relationship is the definition of the healthy family. Urging families to this end is the definition of family therapy.' For transaction to be possible, the individual and the group must be differentiated, not merged. And yet we are still left with a central paradox of human aspiration, spanning all cultures and all ages—that for many, only by losing one's life can life truly be found. It would be too easy simply to dissolve this paradox by some neat resolution. Within the family group as in other social groupings, 'man lives most intensely when he can abandon himself to the system, losing the ("narcissistic") self, even while he is gaining a new, socialised self' (Shands, 1971, p. 22). We cannot and should not try to avoid this strange paradox—for it was not created by the systems theorist and even less so by the family therapist, though both partake in its mystery. Within a wide variety of different contexts the quintessence of relationship is understood as being the union itself, not the parts that make that union possible. The communion of the lover with the beloved one; the union of the mystic with God; the merging of the Zen disciple, in a oneness with the universe; the moment of brief expanded consciousness of the psychedelic experience; the total absorption of the philosopher or scientist in creative thought—for all of these, a loss of self in order to find self is postulated, through the assimilation and identification of the individual with the system to which he happens to belong. 'The ultimate destiny of the human being in search of meaning is thus paradoxically the total identification of the self with the once-alien, the loss of the self in a merging with a system together with others involved in the same loss' (Shands, 1971, p. 23). Perhaps we cannot hope fully to understand, let alone explain, a paradox that has both troubled and enriched the philosophical thought of centuries including that of our own time. We can only consider, reflect and 'ruminate' (to use a favourite word of Shands's) upon its significance for our therapeutic work with families.

Finally, the therapist's basic ideology concerning the value of family life itself, is perhaps the most important factor underlying the way in which he views his work. Some family therapists conceive of their work as helping to support the present somewhat fragile structure of family life, which they feel is being eroded by the pressures of modern Western society. Ackerman (1970b) for example, talks about 'a form of family anomie reflected in a lack of consensus on values' and sees family therapy as 'a force in the community that can give the family new life' (Ackerman, 1971). Others stress a more utilitarian reason for providing family therapy services. They are content to know that, for the present at least, the family exists in Western society, and whilst it sometimes seems to be in rapid decline, there are places where the family is taking on a new sociological importance (Gerson, 1974). While people continue to choose to live in families, it seems reasonable to help them to do so with the maximum amount of fulfilment and the minimum amount of pain. Others again see the family as essentially a malignant and repressive social institution—'an ideological conditioning device' (Cooper, 1971) from which individuals need help in order to break free. Any of these three ideological stances regarding the value of family life are compatible with working as a family therapist.

Partly perhaps because 'the family is the cradle of ambivalence', (Ackerman, 1966b, p. 386) professional workers in other disciplines tend to polarise instantly and fiercely in their reactions to family therapy. 'The challenge of treating a whole family arouses a fiercer rush of ambivalence than any other treatment . . . therapists are either for or against it, with little room for any middle ground.' It is interesting, too, how 'conversion' to either stance is often immediate. 'Friends' and 'opponents' take up their positions, often with surprisingly little evidence upon which to base their decisions. This would again seem to point to the highly charged nature of this method of psychotherapeutic intervention directed towards our primary cradle of emotional experience.

Our need for freedom and autonomy urges us to master 'the system'; to generate revolution; to hasten the death of the family; our need for the compassionate embrace of others—the touch of humanity—restrains us. As human beings we are caught in a dilemma between the inner and the outer. We long to be able to synthesise our need to be separate with our need to be members one of another. My own belief is that the social system which we call the family is essentially neutral in these respects. Often it becomes a strait-jacket, confining its members' aspirations, de-humanising the individuals of which it is composed. But it is also capable of generating the creativity, intimacy and loving acceptance which every man and woman seeks. As therapists, our task is to help make this possible. We all struggle to do so in our different ways, as

Ackerman (1966b, p. 385) the 'grandfather' of family therapy has pointed out:

> In mental healing, there cannot ever be a last word. No form of therapy can be complete in itself. It is rather that each has its own unique potentials; each exerts a selective influence on particular components of pathogenic experience. Each has its own special areas of suitability and effectiveness, also its idiosyncratic weaknesses. It makes little sense, therefore, for therapists to place a vested interest in any single treatment procedure as being elite and better than the others. Let us rather simply admit that each of us prefers to do what each feels he does best.

### Note

1 Some of the difficulties and the advantages of using family therapy in fostering situations are described in a paper entitled 'The use of family sessions in foster home care' in Tod (1971).

# Appendix

Family therapy is being practised by a wide variety of professional workers within the field of mental health. A growing number of agencies too, are devoting considerable resources in terms of staff training and time to the further development of family therapy in this country. The following list describes only a small selection of these agencies. They all offer training facilities to social workers wanting to develop their skills in family therapy.

## I   Department of Mental Health, University of Bristol

Dr Douglas Hooper, Senior Lecturer in Mental Health, is the joint organiser of a psychotherapy training clinic, where conjoint marital therapy is also practised and taught. The training offered by the clinic is postgraduate and is available to professionals within the various fields of mental health, including social work. Dr Hooper is always willing to participate in informal consultations with social workers who are interested in using family therapy in some of their clinical work.

Dr Douglas Hooper,
Senior Lecturer in Mental Health,
Department of Mental Health,
University of Bristol,
41 St Michael's Hill,
Bristol, BS2 8DZ.

## II   The Family Institute, Cardiff

The Family Institute is financed and administered by Dr Barnardo's. It was set up to specialise in the practice and teaching of family therapy and it has close links with the N. W. Ackerman Family Institute, New York. The Institute is staffed by an interdisciplinary team, who work from an eclectic theoretical base, derived chiefly from general systems theory. Therapeutic work is conducted at the Institute and in the families' own homes. The Institute runs a student unit for the Central Council for Education and Training in Social Work, and organises courses and study conferences from time to time for professionals in the mental health field, who wish to extend their skills in family therapy. A research project has been set up to examine the effectiveness of different techniques being currently used in this method of work. Members of staff are always glad to enter into informal discussions with social workers and others about the use of family therapy techniques.

Principal Family Therapist,
The Family Institute,
2 Four Elms Road,
Cardiff, CF2 1LE.
Telephone: Cardiff 26584.

## III  The Institute of Group Analysis

Training in marital and family therapy is offered by the Institute of Group Analysis. The Course in Family and Marital Group Work caters for 120 participants, making use of lectures, demonstrations, films, videotaped material, small group workshops and various action techniques in its teaching programme; it takes place on thirty Tuesday afternoons in the academic year, beginning each October. The course is intended for those who are working with families and who wish to develop skills in conjoint family and marital therapy, in groups for children and parents and in relating to community networks. The course is co-ordinated by Dr A. C. R. Skynner, who also provides the basic orientation lectures. For those who wish to continue their study of family therapy, an advanced course is also provided. Both are open to professionals practising in the various fields of social work and mental health.

The Secretary/Administrator,
Institute of Group Analysis,
1 Bickenhall Mansions,
Bickenhall St,
London, W1.

## IV   The Tavistock Institute of Human Relations

Several departments within the Tavistock Clinic offer training in
family therapy, as well as undertaking the treatment of family
groups and marital pairs:

*1   Department for Children and Parents: The Family Programme*
The Family Programme in the Department for Children and Parents
offers an ongoing clinical service to families, plus workshops and
twice-weekly supervision events for its members. An attempt is being
made to combine an initial psychodynamic approach with further
concepts from systems theory and structural family therapy. In
addition, techniques like family sculpting are used to increase the
experimental potential for both therapists and family. Training
positions are open to all disciplines who hold a clinical position in
the Department or who are formally designated trainees or attached
staff.

*2   Adolescent Department: Young People and Their Families
Workshop*   For the treatment of families as groups, usually with
co-therapists, and for research and training in concepts of family
work, using psycho-analytically based methods.
   Membership is open to all disciplines who hold a clinical position
in the Department or who are formally designated trainees or
attached staff in the Tavistock Centre.

*3   Family Therapy: Seminar for Professionally Qualified Social
Workers Currently Engaged in Family Therapy*   The aim is to
study patterns of family interaction and the various models and
techniques of working with families. Methods of assessment of
families and criteria for family therapy as the treatment of choice are
considered and the use of self in family therapy explored. Members'
own case material is used together with videotape, families and other
action techniques.

The Tavistock Institute of Human Relations,
School of Family Psychiatry and Community Mental Health,
Tavistock Centre,
Belsize Lane,
London, NW3 5BA.

## V   Woodberry Down Child Guidance Unit

The clinic is one of the largest ILEA child guidance and assessment
units in London and has a complete range of specialised staff.

During the past twenty years it has developed a community approach, and an interest in treating the whole family emerged quite naturally out of this orientation.

For the past number of years referrals have been examined with a particular reference to the idea of a total family intake procedure, without prior social history. A high proportion of cases are dealt with in this way. A number of different approaches to the family are employed, varying from a single worker with the family, two workers, who may be of the same sex and 'hetero-sexual co-therapy'. Staff at Woodberry Down Clinic have found that it is possible to space out treatment sessions much more widely for families than for individuals, so that intervals of 3-6 weeks are possible. Despite being in a largely socially deprived area, with a comparatively un-sophisticated population, it does not seem to be difficult to engage all the members of a family. While perhaps the most common theoretical background is derived from psycho-analysis there is broad interpretation of this body of knowledge. The emphasis is on interpersonal relations and feelings in the here and now situation.

There is a long tradition of accepting social work students for field placement here. They are given experience of family therapy. In addition, there is currently a Family Therapy Workshop underway, involving representatives from the various disciplines within the clinic and concerning itself with both theoretical and practical aspects.

The Director,
Woodberry Down Child Guidance Unit,
Inner London Education Authority,
John Scott Health Centre,
Green Lanes,
London, N4 2NU.

# Bibliography

This bibliography includes all articles and books referred to in the text, together with some additional reading material. Several text books (as distinct from collections of papers) have recently made their appearance (of which this can be counted one) and the reader's attention is drawn to these books (marked with an asterisk) which attempt to draw together theoretical ideas and techniques of practice from many different writers.

*Family Process*, a multidisciplinary journal of family study, research and treatment keeps the reader abreast of current developments occurring throughout the field of family therapy. It is published quarterly by the Ackerman Family Institute, New York, and the Mental Research Institute, Palo Alto, California and is edited by Dr Donald Bloch, Director of the Ackerman Family Institute, New York.

Ackerman, N. W. (1958), *The Psychodynamics of Family Life*, Basic Books.
Ackerman, N. W. (1959), 'Transference and counter-transference', *Psychoanalysis and the Psychoanalytic Review*, vol. 46, no. 3.
Ackerman, N. W. (1966a), *Treating the Troubled Family*, Basic Books.
Ackerman, N. W. (1966b), 'Family psychotherapy today: some areas of controversy', *Comprehensive Psychiatry*, vol. 7, no. 5.
Ackerman, N. W. (1970a), 'Child participation in family therapy', *Family Process*, vol. 9, no. 4.
Ackerman, N. W. (1970b), 'What happened to the family?', *Mental Hygiene*, vol. 54, no. 3.
Ackerman, N. W. (1971), 'Family healing in a troubled world', *Social Casework*, vol. 52, April.
Ackerman, N. W., Beatman, F. L. and Sherman, S. N. (eds) (1961), *Exploring the Base for Family Therapy*, Family Service Association of America.
Ackerman, N. W., Beatman, F. L. and Sherman, S. N. (eds) (1967), *Expanding Theory and Practice in Family Therapy*, Family Service Association of America.
Ackerman, N. W., Lieb, J. and Pearce, J. (1970), *Family Therapy in Transition*, Little, Brown & Co.
Ackoff, R. L. (1960), 'Systems, organisations and interdisciplinary research', quoted in 'General System Theory—A critical review', in Beishon, J. and Peters, G. (eds), *Systems Behaviour*, Open University Press, 1972.
Ackoff, R. L. (1971), 'Towards a system of systems concepts', reprinted in Beishon, J. and Peters, G. (eds), *Systems Behaviour*, Open University Press, 1972.
Alger, I. (1973), 'Audio-visual techniques in family therapy', in Bloch (1973).
Alger, I. and Hogan, P. (1970), 'The use of videotape recordings in conjoint marital therapy', in Berger, M. M. (ed.) (1970).
Aponte, H. and Hoffman, L. (1973), 'The open door: a structural approach to a family with an anorectic child', *Family Process*, vol. 12, no. 1.
Armistead, N. (ed.) (1974), *Reconstructing Social Psychology*, Penguin Books.

# Bibliography

Armstrong, R. (1971), 'Two concepts: systems and psychodynamics—paradigms in collision?', in Bradt, J. O. and Moynihan, C. J. (eds) (1971).

Azrin, N. H., Naster, B. J. and Jones, R. (1973), 'Reciprocity counselling: a rapid learning-based procedure for marital counselling', *Behaviour Research and Therapy*, Pergamon, vol. II.

Bardill, D. R. and Bevilacqua, J. J. (1964), 'Family interviewing by two caseworkers', *Social Casework*, vol. 15, no. 5, May.

Barnes, G. G. (1973), 'Working with the family group', *Social Work Today*, Issue no. 3, vol. 4, 1973.

Bateson, G., Jackson, D., Haley, J. and Weakland, J. (1956), 'Toward a theory of schizophrenia', in Jackson, D. (ed.) (1968).

Beels, C. and Ferber, A. (1969), 'Family therapy—a view', *Family Process*, vol. 8, no. 2.

Bell, J. E. (1961), 'Family group therapy', *Public Health Monograph 64*, U.S. Dept of Health, Education and Welfare.

Berger, M. M. (ed.) (1970), 'Videotape techniques in psychiatric training and treatment', Bruner/Mazel.

Berne, E. (1968), *Games People Play*, Penguin Books.

Bertalanffy, L. von (1968), 'General system theory', Allen Lane, Penguin Press.

Bertalanffy, L. von (1972), 'General system theory—a critical review', in Beishon, J. and Peters, G. (eds.), *Systems Behaviour*, Open University Press.

Bloch, D. (ed.) (1973), *Techniques of Family Psychotherapy*, Grune & Stratton.

Boszormenyi-Nagy, I. (1970), 'Critical Incidents in the Context of Family Therapy', in Ackerman, N. W., Lieb, J. and Pearce, J. (eds) (1970).

Boszormenyi-Nagy, I. and Framo, J. (eds) (1965), *Intensive Family Therapy*, Harper & Row.

Bowen, M. (1960), 'A family concept of schizophrenia', in Jackson, D. (ed.), *The Etiology of Schizophrenia*, Basic Books.

Bowen, M. (1971), 'The use of family theory in clinical practice', in Haley, J. (ed.) (1971).

Bradt, J. O and Moynihan, C. J. (eds) (1971), *Systems Therapy*, Groome Child Guidance Center, Washington.

Brody, W. (1967), 'Processes of family change', in Ackerman, N. W., Beatman, F. L. and Sherman, S. N. (eds) (1967).

Bruner, J. S. (1964), 'The course of cognitive growth', *American Psychologist*, vol. 19, index A.

Bruner, J. S. and Postman, L. (1949), 'On the perception of incongruity: a paradigm', *Journal of Personality*, vol. 18, no. 18.

Busfield, J. (1974), 'Family ideology and family pathology', in Armistead, N. (ed.) (1974).

Byng-Hall, J. (1973), 'Family myths used as defence in conjoint family therapy', *British Journal of Medical Psychology*, vol. 46, part 3.

Cade, B. (1975), 'Some ideas on family therapy with low socio-economic families', *Social Work Today*, vol. 6, no. 5.

Cannon, W. B. (1939), *The Wisdom of the Body*, W. W. Norton & Co.

Cooper, D. (1971), *The Death of the Family*, Allen Lane.

Cox, M. (1973), 'The group therapy interaction chronogram', *British Journal of Social Work*, vol. 3, no. 2.

Cox, M. (1974), Correspondence, *Group Analysis*, vol. VII, no. 3.

Dicks, H. V. (1967), *Marital Tensions*, Routledge & Kegan Paul.

Duhl, F. J., Kantor, D. and Duhl, B. S. (1973), 'Learning, space and action in family therapy: a primer of sculpture', in Bloch, D. (ed.) (1973).

Eliot, T. S. (1930), 'Ash Wednesday', in *The Complete Poems and Plays of T. S. Eliot*, Faber, 1969.

Eliot, T. S. (1940), *The Cocktail Party*, Faber.

Erikson, E. H. (1968), *Identity, Youth and Crisis*, W. W. Norton & Co.

Ferreira, A. (1963), 'Family myths and homeostasis', *Archives of General Psychiatry*, vol. 9, November.

*Foley, V. D. (1974), *An Introduction to Family Therapy*, Grune & Stratton.

Framo, J. (1965), 'Systematic research on family dynamics', in Boszormenyi-Nagy, I. and Framo, J. (eds) (1965).

Framo, J. (1970), 'Symptoms from a family transactional viewpoint', in Ackerman, N. W., Lieb, J. and Pierce, J. (eds) (1970).

Framo, J. (ed.) (1972), *Family Interaction: A Dialogue between Family Researchers and Family Therapists,* Springer.

Framo, J. (1973), 'Marriage therapy in a couples group', in Bloch, D. (ed.) (1973).

Freud, S. (1909), 'Analysis of a phobia in a five year old boy', *Complete Works,* vol. 10, edited by Strachey, J., Hogarth Press.

Freud, S. (1912), 'Recommendations for physicians on the psychoanalytic method of treatment', in *Collected Papers,* vol. 2, 1924.

Freud, S. (1915), 'The Unconscious', *Complete Works,* vol. 14, edited by Strachey, J., Hogarth Press.

Fulweiler, C. (1967), 'No man's land', in Haley, J. and Hoffman, L. (eds) (1967).

Gerson, M. (1974), 'The family in the kibbutz', *Journal of Child Psychology and Psychiatry,* vol. 15, no. 1.

Glick, I. D. and Haley, J. (1971), *Family Therapy and Research,* Grune & Stratton.

*Glick, I. D. and Hessler, D. R. (1974), *Marital and Family Therapy,* Grune & Stratton.

Goldstein, H. (1973), *Social Work Practice: A Unitary Approach,* University of South Carolina Press.

Group for the Advancement of Psychiatry (1970), *The Field of Family Therapy,* vol. VII, Mental Health Materials Centre, Inc., New York.

Haley, J. (1962), 'Whither family therapy', *Family Process,* vol. 1, no. 1.

Haley, J. (1963), *Strategies of Psychotherapy,* Grune & Stratton.

Haley, J. (ed.) (1971), *Changing Families,* Grune & Stratton.

Haley, J. and Hoffman, L. (eds) (1967), *Techniques of Family Therapy,* Basic Books.

Hall, A. D. and Fagen, R. E. (1956), 'Definition of system', in Bertalanffy, L. von and Rappaport, A. (eds) *General Systems Yearbook I,* Society of General Systems Research.

Hall, J. and Taylor, K. (1971), 'The emergence of Eric: co-therapy in the treatment of a family with a disabled child', *Family Process,* vol. 10, no. 1.

Hawkins, R. P., Peterson, R. F., Schweid, E. and Bijou, S. W. (1971), 'Behaviour therapy in the home—amelioration of problem parent-child relations with the parent in a therapeutic role', in Haley, J. (ed.) (1971).

Howells, J. (1968), *Theory and Practice of Family Psychiatry,* Oliver & Boyd.

Jackson, D. (1963), Foreword to *Strategies of Psychotherapy,* Grune & Stratton.

Jackson, D. (1965), 'Family rules: the marital quid pro quo', *Archives of General Psychiatry,* vol. 12, June.

Jackson, D. (1967), 'Aspects of conjoint family therapy', in Zuk, G. H. and Boszormenyi-Nagy, I. (eds) (1967).

Jackson, D. (ed.) (1968a), *Human Communication, Vol. I: Communication, Family and Marriage,* Science and Behaviour Books.

Jackson, D. (ed.) (1968b), *Human Communication, Vol. II: Therapy, Communication and Change,* Science and Behaviour Books.

Jackson, D. and Weakland, J. (1961), 'Conjoint family therapy: some considerations on theory, technique and results', *Psychiatry,* vol. 24, supplement to no. 2, May.

Johnson, A. M. and Szurek, S. A. (1952), 'The genesis of antisocial acting out in children and adults', *Psychoanalytic Quarterly,* vol. 21.

Jones, H. V. R. and Dowling, E. (1974), 'Small children seen *and* heard in family therapy', unpublished paper, Family Institute, Cardiff.

Jordan, W. (1970), *Client-Worker Transactions,* Routledge & Kegan Paul.

Jordan, W. (1972), *The Social Worker in Family Situations,* Routledge & Kegan Paul.

Kantor, R. E. and Hoffman, L. (1966), 'Brechtian theatre as a model for conjoint therapy', *Family Process,* vol. 5, no. 2.

Kempler, W. (1973), *Principles of Gestalt Family Therapy,* A. S. Joh. Nordahls Trykkeri, Oslo.

Kempler, W. (1975), 'Transcript of day conference conducted at Family Institute, Cardiff', Barnardo's Publications.

Koestler, A. (1964), *The Act of Creation,* Macmillan.

Lacqueur, H. P. (1972), 'Mechanisms of change in multiple family therapy', in Sager, C. J. and Kaplan, H. S. (eds) (1972).

Laing, R. D. (1970), *Knots,* Tavistock Publications.

# Bibliography

Laing, R. D. (1971a), *The Politics of the Family*, Tavistock Publications.

Laing, R. D. (1971b), 'Rules and meta rules', in Laing, R. D. (1971a).

Laing, R. D. (1971c), 'The family and invalidation', in Laing, R. D. (1971a).

Laing, R. D. (1972), 'Family and individual structure', in Lomas, P. (ed.) *The Predicament of the Family*, Hogarth Press.

Laing, R. D. and Esterson, A. (1964), *Sanity, Madness and the Family*, Penguin Books.

Leichter, E. and Schulman, G. L. (1974), 'Multi-family group therapy', *Family Process*, vol. 13, no. 1.

Lewis, H. R. and Streitfeld, H. S. (1970), *Growth Games*, Harcourt Brace Jovanovich.

Liberman, R. P. (1972), 'Behavioural approaches to family and couple therapy', in Sager, C. J. and Kaplan, H. S. (eds) (1972).

Lidz, T. (1974), Foreword to *Marital and Family Therapy*, Grune & Stratton.

Lidz, T., Flech, S. and Cornelison, A. (1965), *Schizophrenia and the Family*, International Universities Press.

Liebowitz, B. and Black, M. (1974), 'The structure of the Ravich Interpersonal Game/Test', *Family Process*, vol. 13, no. 2.

Loewenstein, C. (1974), 'An intake team in action in a social services department', *British Journal of Social Work*, vol. 4, no. 2.

MacGregor, R. (1962), 'Multiple impact psychotherapy with families', *Family Process*, vol. 1, no. 1.

MacGregor, R., Ritchie, A., Serrans, A., Schuster, F., McDonald, E. and Goolishian, H. (1964), *Multiple Impact Therapy with Families*, McGraw-Hill.

Masters, W. and Johnson, V. (1966), *Human Sexual Response*, Little, Brown & Co.

Miller, N. E. (1959), 'Liberalisation of basic S-R concepts: extensions to conflict behaviour, motivation and social learning', in Koch, S. (ed.), *Psychology: A Study of a Science*, vol. II, McGraw-Hill.

Minuchin, S. (1974a), 'Structural family therapy', in Caplan, G. (ed.) *American Handbook of Psychiatry*, vol. III, Basic Books.

Minuchin, S. (1974b), *Families and Family Therapy*, Tavistock Publications.

Minuchin, S., Montalvo, B., Guerney, B. G., Rosman, B. L. and Shumer, F. (1967), *Families of the Slums*, Basic Books.

Montalvo, B. (1973), 'Aspects of live supervision', *Family Process*, vol. 12, no. 4.

Napier, A. Y. and Whitaker, C. (1973), 'Problems of the beginning family therapist', in Bloch, D. (ed.) (1973).

Naranjo, C. (1970), 'Present-centredness: technique, prescription and ideal', in Fagan, J. and Shepherd, I. L. (eds) (1970), *Gestalt Therapy Now*, Science and Behaviour Books.

North, M. (1972), *The Secular Priests: Psychotherapists in Contemporary Society*, Allen & Unwin.

Olson, D. H. (1970), 'Marital and family therapy: integrative review and critique', *Journal of Marriage and the Family*, vol. 32.

Papp, P., Silverstein, O. and Carter, E. (1973), 'Family sculpting in preventive work with "well families"', *Family Process*, vol. 12, no. 2.

Pearlstein, S. (1973), 'Beginning family therapy', in *Family Therapy in Social Work*, Family Welfare Association, Conference Papers.

Pearson, G. (1974), 'Prisons of love: the reification of the family in family therapy', in Armistead, N. (ed.) (1974).

Pincus, L. (1971), 'The nature of marital interaction', in *The Marital Relationship as a Focus for Casework*, Tavistock Institute of Human Relations.

Pittman, F. S. (1973), 'Managing acute psychiatric emergencies', in Bloch, D. (ed.) (1973).

Pittman, F. S., Flomenhaft, K. and De Young, C. (1967), 'Cleaning house', in Haley, J. and Hoffman, L. (eds) (1967).

Ransom, D. (1972), Review of 'The war with words', by Shands, H. C., *Family Process*, vol. 11, no. 3.

Ravich, R. (1969), 'Game-testing in conjoint marital psychotherapy', *American Journal of Psychotherapy*, vol. 23, no. 2.

Reichard, S. and Tillman, C. (1950), 'Patterns of parent-child relationships in schizophrenia', *Psychiatry*, vol. 13, no. 2.

Reiss, D. (1971), 'Varieties of consensual experience, I—A theory for relating family interaction to individual thinking', *Family Process*, vol. 10, no. 1.

Rice, D. G., Fey, W. F. and Kepecs, J. C. (1972), 'Therapist experience and "style" as factors in co-therapy', *Family Process*, vol. 11, no. 1.

Richter, H. E. (1974), *The Family as Patient*, Souvenir Press.

Riskin, J. M and Faunce, E. E. (1972), 'An evaluative review of family interaction research', *Family Process*, vol. 11, no. 4.

Roberts, W. L. (1968), 'Working with the family group in a child guidance clinic', *British Journal of Psychiatric Social Work*, vol. 9, no. 4.

Rosenbaum, M. (1970), 'The issues of privacy and privileged communication', in Berger, M. M. (ed.) (1970).

Rubinstein, D. and Weiner, O. R. (1967), 'Co-therapy teamwork relationships in family therapy', in Zuk, G. H. and Boszormenyi-Nagy, I. (eds) (1967).

Sager, C. J. and Kaplan, H. S. (eds) (1972), *Progress in Group and Family Therapy* Bruner/Mazel.

Sartre, J. P. (1964), *Words*, Hamilton.

Satir, V. (1964), *Conjoint Family Therapy*, Science and Behaviour Books.

Satir, V. (1972), *People-Making*, Science and Behaviour Books.

Searles, H. (1959), 'The effort to drive the other person crazy—an element in the aetiology and psychotherapy of schizophrenia', *British Journal of Medical Psychology*, vol. 32, part 1.

Shands, H. C. (1971), *The War with Words: Structure and Transcendence*, Mouton, The Hague.

Simon, R. M. (1972), 'Sculpting the family', *Family Process*, vol. 11, no. 1.

Skynner, A. C. R. (1969a), 'A group-analytic approach to conjoint family therapy', *Journal of Child Psychiatry and Psychology*, vol. 10.

Skynner, A. C. R. (1969b), 'Indications and contra-indications for conjoint family therapy', *International Journal of Social Psychiatry*, vol. 15, no. 4.

Skynner, A. C. R. (1971), 'The minimum sufficient network', *Social Work Today*, vol. 2, no. 9.

Skynner, A. C. R. (1974), 'Boundaries', *Social Work Today*, vol. 5, no. 10.

Slipp, S., Ellis, S. and Kressel, K. (1974), 'Factors associated with engagement in family therapy', *Family Process*, vol. 13, no. 4.

Soloman, M. (1969), 'Family therapy dropouts: resistance to change', *Canadian Psychiatric Association Journal*, vol. 14.

Soloman, M. (1973), 'A developmental, conceptual premise for family therapy', *Family Process*, vol. 12, no. 2.

Sonne, J., Speck, R. V., Jungreis, J. E. (1962), 'The absent member manoeuvre as a resistance in family therapy of schizophrenia', *Family Process*, vol. 1, no. 1.

Sonne, J. and Lincoln, G. (1965), 'Heterosexual co-therapy team experiences during family therapy', *Family Process*, vol. 4, no. 2.

Speck, R. V. and Attneave, C. L. (1971), 'Social network intervention', in Haley, J. (ed.) (1971).

Speck, R. V. and Attneave, C. L. (1973), *Family Networks*, Pantheon Books.

Speer, D. C. (1970), 'Family systems: morphostasis and morphogenesis or "Is homeostasis enough?"', *Family Process*, vol. 9, no. 3.

Spitzer, S. P, Swanson, R. M. and Lehr, R. K. (1968), 'Audience reactions and careers of psychiatric patients', *Family Process*, vol. 8, no. 2.

Stoller, F. H. (1970), 'Videotape feedback in the marathon and encounter group', in Berger, M. M. (ed.) (1970).

Tod, R. (1971), *Social Work in Foster Care*, Longman.

Traux, C. B. and Carkhuff, R. B. (1967), *Toward Effective Counseling and Psychotherapy: Teaching and Practice*, Aldine.

Walrond-Skinner, S. (1974), 'Training for family therapy', *Social Work Today*, vol. 5, no. 5.

Watermann, C. E. (1971), 'Counter-transference in family therapy', in Bradt, J. O. and Moynihan, C. J. (eds) (1971).

Watzlawick, P., Beavin, A. B. and Jackson, D. (1968), *The Pragmatics of Human Communication*, Faber.

Weakland, J., Fisch, R., Watzlawick, P. and Bodin, A. M. (1974), 'Brief therapy: focused problem resolution', *Family Process*, vol. 13, no. 2.

Wells, R. A., Dilkes, T. C. and Trivelli, N. (1972), 'The results of family therapy: a critical review of the literature', *Family Process*, vol. 11, no. 2.

# Bibliography

Wertheim, E. S. (1973), 'Family unit therapy and the science and typology of family systems', *Family Process,* vol. 12, no. 4.

Whitaker, C. A. (1967), 'The growing edge', in Haley, J. and Hoffman, L. (eds) (1967).

Whitaker, C. A. (1972), 'A longitudinal view of therapy styles where N = 1', Critique of the Rice, Fey and Kepecs article, *Family Process,* vol. 11, no. 1.

Whitaker, C. A., Felder, R. E. and Warkentin, J. (1965), 'Counter transference in the family treatment of schizophrenia', in Boszormenyi-Nagy, I. and Framo, J. (eds) (1965).

Wynne, L. (1965), 'Some indications and contra-indications for exploratory family therapy', in Boszormenyi-Nagy, I. and Framo, J. (eds) (1965).

Wynne, L., Ryckoff, I. M., Day, J. and Hirsch, S. I. (1958), 'Pseudo-mutuality in the family relations of schizophrenics', *Psychiatry,* vol. 21, no. 2.

Yalom, I. D. (1970), *The Theory and Practice of Group Psychotherapy,* Basic Books.

Zilbach, J. J., Bergel, E. and Gass, C. (1972), 'The role of the young child in family therapy', in Sager, C. J. and Kaplan, H. S. (eds) (1972).

Zuk, G. H. (1971), 'Family therapy', in Haley, J. (ed.) (1971).

Zuk, G. H. and Boszormenyi-Nagy, I. (eds) (1967) *Family Therapy and Disturbed Families,* Science and Behaviour Books.